THE CLINICAL LABORATORY MANUAL SERIES:

Urinalysis

Other Delmar titles in this Clinical Laboratory Manual Series include:

Dean/Whitlock: The Clinical Laboratory Manual Series: Clinical Chemistry
Hoeltke: The Clinical Laboratory Manual Series: Phlebotomy
Marshall: The Clinical Laboratory Manual Series: Microbiology
Russell: The Clinical Laboratory Manual Series: Hematology
Smith: The Clinical Laboratory Manual Series: Immunology
Whitlock: The Clinical Laboratory Manual Series: Immunohematology

Also available from Delmar Publishers:

Davis: Phlebotomy: A Client-Based Approach
Fong/Lakomia: Microbiology for Health Careers, 5E
Hoeltke: The Complete Textbook of Phlebotomy
Marshall: Fundamental Skills for the Clinical Laboratory Professional
Walters: Basic Medical Laboratory Techniques, 3E

THE CLINICAL LABORATORY MANUAL SERIES:

Urinalysis

John C. Flynn Jr., Ph.D., M.S., MT(ASCP)SBB
Sheryl A. Whitlock, M.A., MT(ASCP)BB

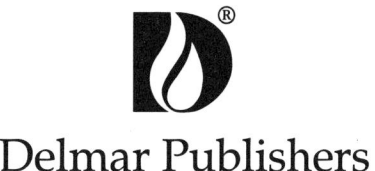

Delmar Publishers

an International Thomson Publishing company I(T)P®

Albany • Bonn • Boston • Cincinnati • Detroit • London • Madrid
Melbourne • Mexico City • New York • Pacific Grove • Paris • San Francisco
Singapore • Tokyo • Toronto • Washington

NOTICE TO THE READER

Publisher does not warrant or guarantee any of the products described herein or perform any independent analysis in connection with any of the product information contained herein. Publisher does not assume, and expressly disclaims, any obligation to obtain and include information other than that provided to it by the manufacturer.

The reader is expressly warned to consider and adopt all safety precautions that might be indicated by the activities described herein and to avoid all potential hazards. By following the instructions contained herein, the reader willingly assumes all risks in connection with such instructions.

The publisher makes no representation or warranties of any kind, including but not limited to, the warranties of fitness for particular purpose or merchantability, nor are any such representations implied with respect to the material set forth herein, and the publisher takes no responsibility with respect to such material. The publisher shall not be liable for any special, consequential, or exemplary damages resulting, in whole or part, from the readers' use of, or reliance upon, this material.

Delmar Publishers' Online Services

To access Delmar on the World Wide Web, point your browser to:

http://www.delmar.com/delmar.html

To access through Gopher: gopher://gopher.delmar.com

(Delmar Online is part of "thomson.com", an Internet site with information on more than 30 publishers of the International Thomson Publishing organization.)
For information on our products and services:
email: info@delmar.com
or call 800-347-7707

Cover Design: joanne beckmann design

Delmar Staff
Publisher: Susan Simpfenderfer
Acquisitions Editor: Marion Waldman
Project Editor: William Trudell
Art and Design Coordinator: Rich Killar
Production Coordinator: John Mickelbank
Editorial Assistant: Sarah Holle
Marketing Manager: Darryl L. Caron

COPYRIGHT © 1997
By Delmar Publishers
a division of International Thomson Publishing Inc.

The ITP logo is a trademark under license.

Printed in the United States of America

For more information, contact:

Delmar Publishers
3 Columbia Circle, Box 15015
Albany, New York 12212-5015

International Thomson Editores
Campos Eliseos 385, Piso 7
Col Polanco
11560 Mexico D F Mexico

International Thomson Publishing Europe
Berkshire House 168-173
High Holborn
London, WC1V 7AA
England

International Thomson Publishing GmbH
Konigswinterer Strasse 418
53227 Bonn
Germany

Thomas Nelson Australia
102 Dodds Street
South Melbourne, 3205
Victoria Australia

International Thomson Publishing Asia
221 Henderson Road
#05-10 Henderson Building
Singapore 0315

Nelson Canada
1120 Birchmount Road
Scarborough, Ontario
Canada, M1K 5G4

International Thomson Publishing–Japan
Hirakawacho Kyowa Builidng, 3F
2-2-1 Hirakawacho
Chiyoda-ku, Tokyo 102
Japan

All rights reserved. No part of this work covered by the copyright hereon may be reproduced or used in any form or by any means—graphic, electronic, or mechanical, including photocopying, recording, taping, or information storage and retrieval systems—without the written permission of the publisher.

1 2 3 4 5 6 7 8 9 10 XXX 02 01 00 99 98 97 96

Library of Congress Cataloging-in-Publication Data

Flynn, John C., 1958–
    Urinalysis / John C. Flynn, Sheryl Whitlock.
      p. cm.—(Clinical laboratory manual series)
    Includes bibliographical references and index.
    ISBN 0-8273-7196-9
    1. Urine—Analysis—Laboratory manuals. I. Whitlock, Sheryl. II. Title. III. Series.
    [DNLM: 1. Urinalysis—laboratory manuals. 2. Urinalysis—problems. QY 25 F648u 1997]
RB53.F67 1997
616.07'566—dc20
DNLM/DLC
for Library of Congress   96-2564
                                                          CIP

ACKNOWLEDGMENTS

Special thanks for their assistance in preparing this manual is extended to the following persons:

Theresa Dean, MT(ASCP)
Montgomery County Community College
Blue Bell, Pennsylvania

Linda Pileggi
Montgomery County Community College
Blue Bell, Pennsylvania

CONTENTS

List of Laboratory Exercises *ix*
Preface *xi*

UNIT 1 **Formation of Urine** *1*
Introduction *3*
Composition of Urine *3*
Renal Structure *3*
Renal Physiology and Urine Formation *6*
Summary *11*
Review Questions *11*

UNIT 2 **Quality Control and Safety in the Urinalysis Laboratory** *13*
Introduction *15*
Quality Control in the Urinalysis Laboratory *15*
Safety in the Urinalysis Laboratory *18*
Summary *24*
Review Questions *24*

UNIT 3 **Specimen Collection** *26*
Introduction *28*
Specimen Containers and Labeling *28*
Types of Specimens *28*
Preservatives *31*
Summary *32*
Review Questions *33*

UNIT 4 **Physical Examination of Urine** *35*
Introduction *37*
Color *37*
Appearance *38*
Specific Gravity *38*
Odor *41*
Summary *43*
Review Questions *43*
Further Activities *44*

UNIT 5 **Chemical Examination of Urine** *45*
Introduction *47*
Reagent Strips *47*
Confirmatory and Supplementary Tests *56*
Instrumentation *58*
Summary *60*
Review Questions *61*

Contents

UNIT 6 **Microscopic Examination of Urine** *63*
Introduction *65*
Use of the Microscope *65*
Microscopic Examination of Urine *71*
Summary *86*
Review Questions *86*

UNIT 7 **Case Studies in Urinalysis** *88*
Introduction *88*
Case Study Number 1 *89*
Case Study Number 2 *90*
Case Study Number 3 *91*
Case Study Number 4 *92*
Case Study Number 5 *93*
Case Study Number 6 *94*
Case Study Number 7 *95*
Case Study Number 8 *96*
Case Study Number 9 *97*
Case Study Number 10 *98*
Summary *99*

Appendix A **Answers to Review Questions** *100*
Appendix B **Answers to Case Studies** *101*
References *103*
Index *105*

LIST OF LABORATORY EXERCISES

UNIT 1
Exercise 1: Cellular Components of Urine *4*
Exercise 2: Diagramming a Nephron *6*
Exercise 3: Active and Passive Reabsorption *8*
Exercise 4: Countercurrent Mechanism *9*
Exercise 5: ADH and Aldosterone *10*
Exercise 6: Physiologic Functions of the Nephron *10*

UNIT 2
Exercise 7: Use of Lyophilized Controls *16*
Exercise 8: Analysis of Urine Control Values *17*
Exercise 9: Handwashing Techniques *19*
Exercise 10: Biohazard Protection *20*
Exercise 11: Removal of Soiled Gloves *20*
Exercise 12: Safety Procedure *21*
Exercise 13: MSDS Sheets *22*
Exercise 14: NFPA Labels *23*
Exercise 15: Location of Safety Equipment *23*

UNIT 3
Exercise 16: Urine Containers *29*
Exercise 17: Clean Catch Midstream Procedure *30*
Exercise 18: Urine Specimens *31*
Exercise 19: Urine Preservatives *32*

UNIT 4
Exercise 20: Urine Collection *38*
Exercise 21: Urine Appearance *39*
Exercise 22: Calculating Specific Gravity *40*
Exercise 23: Comparing the Urinometer and Refractometer *42*

UNIT 5
Exercise 24: Chemical Reagent Strips *48*
Exercise 25: False-Positive and False-Negative Reactions *55*
Exercise 26: Chemical Tests *55*
Exercise 27: Urinary Chemical Testing *56*
Exercise 28: Investigating Confirmatory Tests *58*
Exercise 29: Confirmatory Testing *59*
Exercise 30: Urinalysis Instrumentation *60*

UNIT 6
Exercise 31: Determination of Magnification *67*
Exercise 32: Identification of Microscope Parts *68*
Exercise 33: Use of the Microscope *69*
Exercise 34: Storage of the Microscope *71*
Exercise 35: Comparison of Types of Microscopy *73*
Exercise 36: Reporting Microscopic Urinalysis *84*
Exercise 37: Microscopic Examination of Urine *84*

PREFACE

By John C. Flynn, Jr. and Sheryl Whitlock

The *Clinical Laboratory Manual Series* is designed for use by instructors in vocational schools, community colleges, and the clinical laboratory environment. Its purpose is to give the medical laboratory technician the best training possible to keep up with the demands of the rapidly changing health care environment. Safety issues are strongly emphasized in all manuals.

The *Urinalysis Manual* of this series emphasizes a hands-on approach to learning. Exercises are included throughout this manual to provide the learner with practice and feedback to enhance the learning experience.

Urinalysis is an area of the laboratory that is frequently a section of either Hematology or Clinical Chemistry. Technicians in the department perform the urinalysis testing as a part of the daily test load. Education in the urinalysis procedure is important to the success of the technician working in the laboratory. Results obtained during urinalysis provide the clinician with useful information for diagnosis and treatment of their patients.

The emphasis on safety is one feature of this manual. The student needs to adopt these safety practices as a part of the testing process. Universal precautions have been outlined and included in all procedures with potential biohazard exposure. Clinical sites and laboratories will use the safe practices incorporated in this manual as protection from accidental exposure to biohazardous materials. Quality control emphasis, as well as exercises, is included in the text. This information provides the technician with an understanding of monitoring test practices to assure the clinician of accurate test results.

Each unit includes learning objectives, boldfaced terms found in a glossary, and review questions. The topics discussed include specimen collection, and physical, chemical, and microbiological testing of urines. Case studies are provided in Unit 7 to provide the student with application of the material included in the preceding units. These case studies reflect the clinical conditions discussed in conjunction with testing protocol.

This manual is intended to serve as a compilation of information designed to provide the learner with an overview of urinalysis testing processes. Additionally, common clinical conditions and how test results will be reflected in these clinical states are addressed. In summation, this manual is designed to provide information that will not only educate the learner, but also improve patient care.

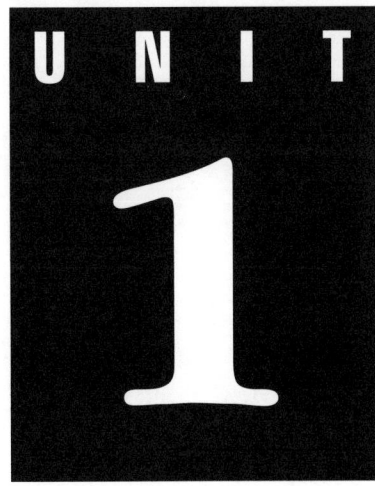

Formation of Urine

LEARNING OBJECTIVES

After studying this unit, it is the responsibility of the student to know the following objectives:

- Define all terms in the glossary.

- Identify the parts of the kidney on a diagram and state the function of each.

- Trace a path of urine formation through the kidney.

- Describe major physiologic functions the kidney employs during urine formation.

- Outline how kidney function affects acid-base balance of the body.

- Describe the effects of ADH and aldosterone on urine formation.

- Describe the composition of urine to include substances eliminated via the urine.

- List factors that affect the concentration of solutes in urine.

- Unit 1

GLOSSARY

Bowman's capsule a two-layered cellular envelope that surrounds the tuft of capillaries known as the glomerulus in the nephron.

calyx (plural calyces) the portion of the renal pelvis which receives forming urine from the collecting tubules and pools that forming urine.

collecting tubule the portion of the nephron into which the distal convoluted tubules pool the urine; this tubule will then pool the urine into the calyces.

concentration to increase the strength by removal of water.

cortex the outer layer of the kidney; contains glomeruli and convoluted tubules.

countercurrent fluid flow and exchange of water and electrolytes occurring in opposite directions as urine passes through the loop of Henle.

distal convoluted tubule the twisted portion of the nephron which is found following the loop of Henle and prior to the collecting tubule.

fenestrated with one or more openings.

filtration passage through a material that will only allow certain substances to move to the other side.

glomerulus a tuft of capillaries found at the beginning of each nephron.

hypertonic having an osmotic pressure greater than the comparison fluid.

loop of Henle the U-shaped tubule which connects the proximal and distal convoluted tubules in the nephron; consists of descending and ascending limbs plus a hairpin-shaped turn.

medulla the inner portion of the kidney which includes collecting tubules.

nephron the functional and structural unit of the kidney which is the primary urine producing unit.

peritoneum a membrane which lines the abdominal and pelvic cavities.

proximal convoluted tubule a portion of the nephron which follows Bowman's capsule and precedes the loop of Henle; consists of a twisted section of tubule.

reabsorption to absorb again after having been secreted.

renal pelvis a portion of the kidney; an upper portion of the ureter into which the renal calyces empty.

renal threshold the plasma concentration of a substance which will allow that substance to begin to be excreted into the urine.

secretion to release a substance into a separate area from its origination.

ultrafiltrate liquid produced by filtration of the plasma at Bowman's capsule; produces the fluid which will ultimately become urine.

Formation of Urine

INTRODUCTION

Testing of urine has historically been one of the mainstays on the menu of available laboratory tests. Gross examination of urine for smell, color, and even taste has been used for centuries to aid in the determination of the clinical condition and metabolic status of the patient. Urine testing has been expanded to include chemical tests that help determine renal function status. In addition, urine can be utilized to perform analyses for toxicology, drugs of abuse, therapeutic drug levels, and microbiological cultures. Historically, the routine urinalysis was the front runner to all of these additional tests. Routine urinalysis is still frequently performed as a part of physical examinations, screening for metabolic abnormalities, and preoperative profiles. To understand the significance of urinalysis, it is vital to understand renal structure and function as well as urine formation.

COMPOSITION OF URINE

The primary constituent of urine is water. Urine is an **ultrafiltrate** of plasma, consisting of approximately 95% water with solutes dissolved in the liquid. The actual concentration of the solutes varies with factors such as hydration state of the body, diet, exercise, and general health. The solutes in highest concentration are summarized in Table 1.1.

Substances which are not solutes, but are cellular, are also found in urine. These cellular items are summarized in Table 1.1. Quantities of cellular components vary depending on the sex, physical status, and state of hydration of the patient. When found in sufficient quantities, these cellular items may indicate clinical conditions or infections.

RENAL STRUCTURE

The kidneys are a pair of organs located on either side of the spinal column, behind the **peritoneum**, and against the muscles of the back. Each organ is shaped like a bean and surrounded by a fibrous capsule. Underneath this capsule are two major layers. These layers are the **cortex** and the **medulla**, consecutively (see Figure 1.1).

Table 1.1. Urinary Constituents

Solutes	Cellular Components
Urea	Epithelial cells
Chloride	Blood cells
Sodium	Bacteria
Potassium	Yeast
Ammonia	Mucus
Creatinine	Crystals
	Uric acid

• Unit 1

E X E R C I S E **EXAMINING URINALYSIS REPORT FORMS**

In small groups, students should be provided with sample report forms used for urinalysis in a clinical laboratory. Each group should do the following:

1. Look briefly at the report forms to become familiar with the items reported.
2. Using the report form, determine the normal levels of cellular items found in the urine.
3. Determine the system used to report chemical and cellular items.
4. Create several fictitious reports with results of the urinalysis.
5. Role play phone reports of urinalysis.

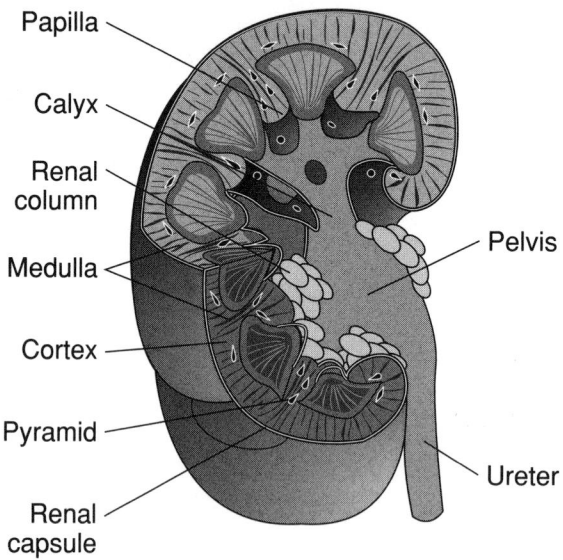

fig. 1.1. Cross section of the kidney.

The cortex contains the major parts of the functional units of the kidney. The **nephron** is this functional unit (see Figure 1.2). Each kidney contains more than a million urine-forming nephrons. The individual nephron is a microscopic unit which begins in the cortex. It begins with a cluster of capillaries called the **glomerulus**. These capillaries are surrounded by a layer of epithelial cells called **Bowman's capsule**. Bowman's capsule is a cup-shaped structure that serves as the beginning of the tubular system of the nephron. It is here that filtering of the blood occurs. Bowman's capsule opens into the **proximal convoluted tubule**, that straightens out into a structure called the **loop of Henle**. The loop of Henle

Formation of Urine

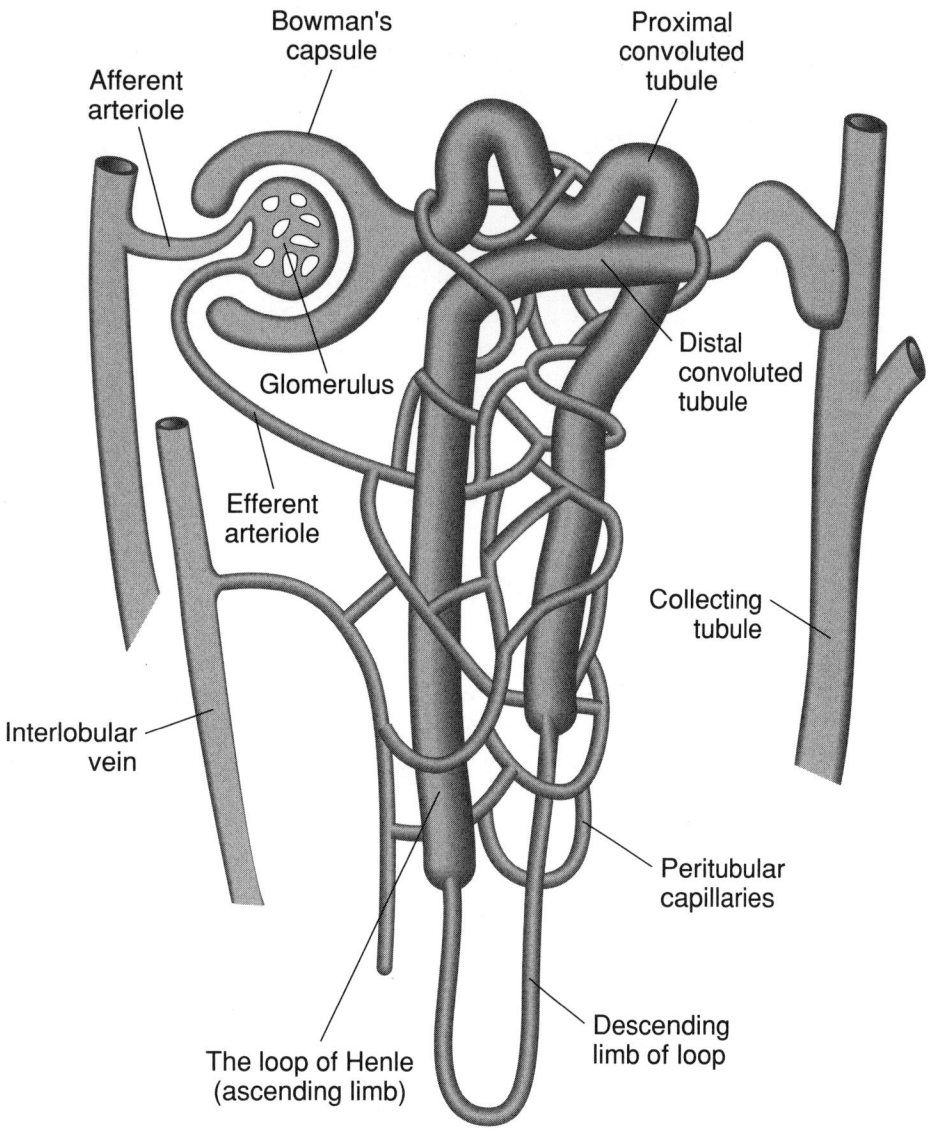

fig. 1.2. A single nephron unit.

is shaped similar to a hairpin. It originates with a descending limb which extends into the medulla where it transforms into the U-shaped turn and becomes the ascending limb. The ascending limb extends into the cortex and connects to the **distal convoluted tubule**. Two or more distal convoluted tubules merge to form the **collecting tubule** or duct of the nephron which extends back into the medulla. Once the urine has formed in the nephrons, it passes into the **renal pelvis** by way of the collecting tubules (Figure 1.1). Each collecting tubule empties, along with others, into a collecting area called a **calyx**. These calyces merge to form larger areas until the renal pelvis is formed (Figure 1.1). The renal pelvis is the major collecting area for urine. From the renal pelvis, the urine flows into the ureter and passes through the remainder of the urinary tract.

• Unit 1

EXERCISE 2: DIAGRAMMING A NEPHRON

Individually or in small groups, the students should complete the following activities:

1. Using colored pencils or pens, diagram a nephron.
2. Identify individual parts with different colors.
3. Using arrows, trace the path of urine formation through the nephron.

RENAL PHYSIOLOGY AND URINE FORMATION

With regard to urine formation, the four basic physiologic functions of the kidney are **filtration, concentration, reabsorption,** and **secretion**. These functions occur at specific places in the nephron, and more than one function may take place concurrently. These functions are summarized in Table 1.2.

FILTRATION

Urine formation begins with filtration. The glomerulus provides an area of blood flow that enables the tubular system to filter materials from the blood. The glomerulus is composed of **fenestrated** capillaries that permit filtration but will not allow passage of large molecules or blood cells. As blood passes through the capillaries, the epithelial cells of Bowman's capsule filter out materials with molecular weights of less than 70,000 daltons. A plasma ultrafiltrate, produced as a result of filtration, is the beginning of urine formation. This ultrafiltrate passes into the proximal convoluted tubule where metabolic functions begin. Because the filtration in the glomerulus is nonspecific, certain substances are removed in higher concentrations than desirable for maintenance of some of the body's metabolic systems. To prevent an imbalance, some substances are returned to the plasma from the ultrafiltrate. For this reason, the processes of reabsorption and secretion take place beginning in the proximal convoluted tubule.

Table 1.2. Kidney Functions

Function	Location
Filtration	Glomerulus
Reabsorption	Entire nephron except the ascending loop of Henle
Secretion	Proximal convoluted tubule
Concentration	Distal convoluted tubule
	Loop of Henle

Formation of Urine

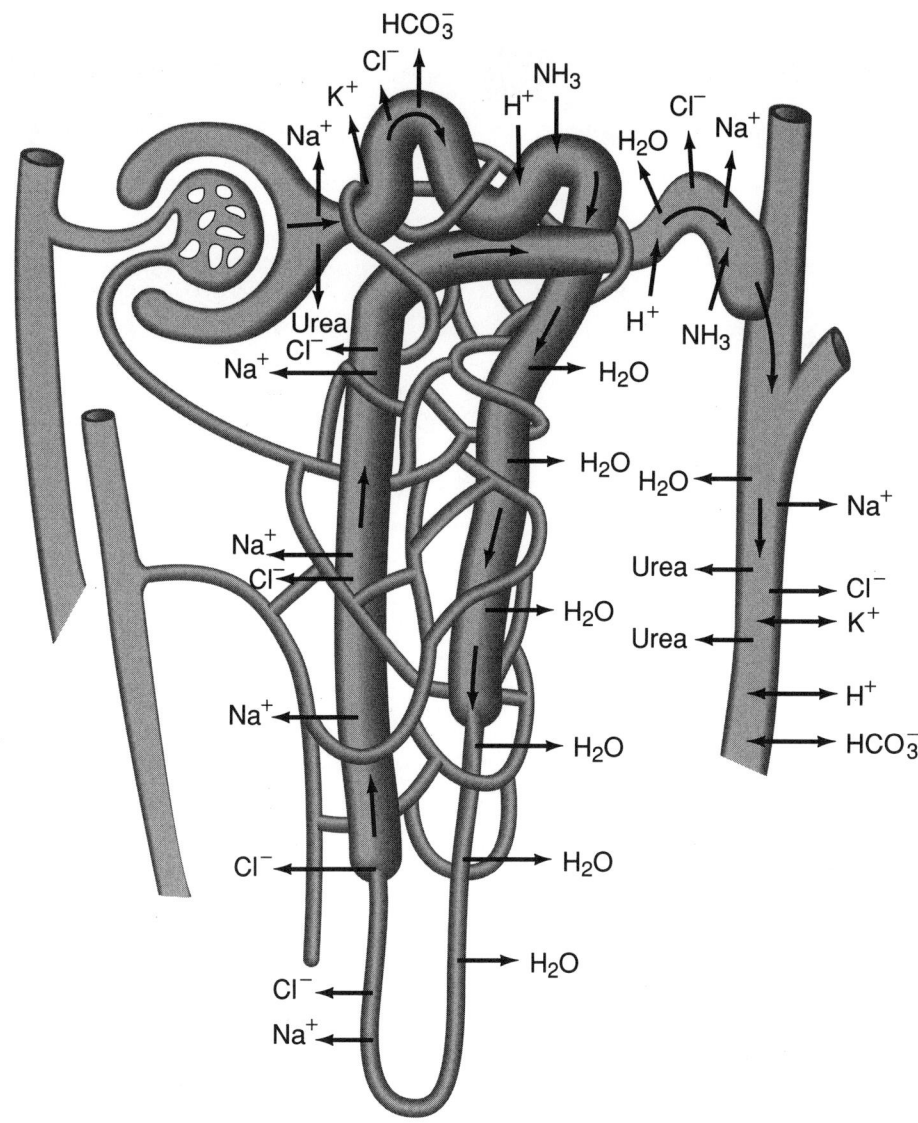

fig. 1.3. Absorption and secretion within the nephron unit.

REABSORPTION

Reabsorption occurs across the membrane of the tubule and uses the mechanisms of active and passive transport. Reabsorption of water occurs passively throughout the nephron with the exception of the ascending loop of Henle (see Figure 1.3). Passive transport in the tubule is responsible for the reabsorption of water, chloride, potassium, and urea. During passive reabsorption, the movement of molecules is due to differences in salt concentration gradients on either side of the membrane.

Active transport results in reabsorption of glucose, sodium, bicarbonate, amino acids, proteins, uric acid, magnesium, calcium, phosphate, and other substances. Active transport requires energy and a carrier protein. Unlike passive mechanisms, active transport occurs across concentration gradients and is affected by high levels of the substances being reabsorbed. When the plasma

• Unit 1

EXERCISE 3 ACTIVE AND PASSIVE REABSORPTION

Individually or in small groups the students should perform the following activities:

1. Diagram the loop of Henle.
2. Label the diagram.
3. On the diagram, identify substances being reabsorbed. Use different color arrows for active and passive reabsorption.
4. Compare the diagram with another student in the group.

concentration exceeds the level that the tubules can contain, the substance will begin to appear in the urine. The **renal threshold** is said to have been exceeded.

SECRETION

The process of secretion occurs with reabsorption in the proximal and distal convoluted tubules. This helps to eliminate foreign and toxic substances from the circulation and maintain acid-base balance by secretion of hydrogen ions.

Substances eliminated from the body by the urine include those not normally found in the body, substances not fully metabolized, and those bound to a carrier protein. Examples are summarized in Table 1.3.

Acid-Base Balance. Acid-base balance is a function of the kidney and involves three mechanisms for the transport of hydrogen ions. The first mechanism aids in acid-base balance by preventing the loss of bicarbonate. Bicarbonate is a vital part of the blood buffering system. Loss through the urine must be minimized. This is accomplished by tubular secretion of hydrogen ions in the proximal convoluted tubule. After secretion, hydrogen combines with available bicarbonate to form H_2O and CO_2. Carbon dioxide diffuses into the cells, where it is converted back into bicarbonate and retained for use by the body (Figure 1.3).

The second and third mechanisms for hydrogen secretion are used to maintain the body at the proper pH. This is accomplished by secretion of excess hydrogen through the urine. In the proximal convoluted tubule, the hydrogen

Table 1.3. Substances Eliminated Through the Urine

- Drugs
  Penicillin
  Salicylate
- Radiographic contrast media
- Mannitol
- Thiamine
- Unconjugated bilirubin

Formation of Urine

ions combine with phosphates and are excreted in the urine. A similar method is used in the distal convoluted tubule where ammonia is secreted. The excess hydrogen secreted in the proximal convoluted tubule combines with the secreted ammonia and is excreted in the urine. These three processes occur concurrently and help to maintain the acid-base balance of the body.

CONCENTRATION

The final physiologic mechanism is concentration. As the filtrate leaves the proximal convoluted tubule, the concentration process begins to intensify. The majority of the concentration phase occurs after the urine leaves the proximal convoluted tubule and passes into the loop of Henle. It continues in the distal convoluted tubule.

During the filtration process, the amount of water filtered into the ultrafiltrate is greater than that lost in the urine. Because the renal medulla is **hypertonic**, water will passively leave the tubule as the urine flows through the descending limb of the loop of Henle. Salts will not flow across the gradient or be reabsorbed. As the fluid passes into the ascending limb of the loop of Henle, the sodium and chloride will be reabsorbed, while the amount of water will remain constant within the tube (Figure 1.3). This results from the impermeability of the tubule wall to water.

The reabsorption process occurring in the loops is known as a **countercurrent** process. It is the countercurrent nature of this process that helps to keep the osmotic gradient constant within the medulla and accounts for the concentration of the formed urine when it reaches the collecting tubule.

As the filtrate leaves the ascending limb, it enters the distal convoluted tubule for the final phase of concentration. Reabsorption and secretion aid in the concentration process. Reabsorption of water is dependent on antidiuretic hormone (ADH) and the osmotic gradient. The hormone ADH controls the permeability of the tubule walls to water. When the level of the hormone is high, more water is reabsorbed and the urine will be concentrated. Working in conjunction with

---

EXERCISE **COUNTERCURRENT MECHANISM**

Individually or in small groups, the students should complete the following activities:

1. Diagram the loop of Henle.
2. Indicate the countercurrent mechanism on the diagram.
3. Label the substances reabsorbed and secreted. Place the absorbed and secreted substances on the appropriate area of the diagram where the activity is *happening*.
4. In small groups discuss how the urine will be affected if the countercurrent mechanism is not working properly.

- Unit 1

ADH is aldosterone. Aldosterone works in combination with ADH and causes the increase of sodium absorption and potassium secretion.

As urine leaves the distal convoluted tubule, it enters the collecting tubule, which is also under the control of ADH and aldosterone. The collecting tubule aids in the final concentration of the urine before its passage into the calyces and subsequently through the remaining urinary tract.

EXERCISE 5 ADH AND ALDOSTERONE

Working in small groups, the students should research ADH and aldosterone. The references may be provided by the instructor or assigned readings in a library. The students should identify the following information and produce a chart to share with the class.

1. The organ of origin of ADH and aldosterone.
2. Physiological functions of each hormone.
3. Disease states which cause increases and decreases in these hormones.
4. How abnormalities in the levels of each hormone will affect the final urine.

The researched information should be shared with the class.

EXERCISE 6 PHYSIOLOGIC FUNCTIONS OF THE NEPHRON

Each student should complete the following:

1. Make a diagram of a nephron.
2. Label each part of the nephron.
3. Label each part with the metabolic function using the following markings:
   F = filtration
   C = concentration
   R = reabsorption
   S = secretion
4. Have the instructor check the work.

Formation of Urine

SUMMARY

Testing of urine and examination of its constituents play a major part in establishing the metabolic state of an individual. The composition of urine varies not only with clinical conditions but also during the fluctuations in hydration during the course of a day. Cellular components may be significant in establishing or confirming a clinical diagnosis.

Understanding the formation of urine and its composition will be useful in understanding the process of urinalysis and interpretation of the results when performing the tests. The nephron is vital to the formation of urine. Understanding the structure and function of the parts of the nephron adds to the full comprehension of urine formation. Material presented in this unit will be used in future units as a basis for understanding concepts.

REVIEW QUESTIONS

1. The microscopic unit that carries out the filtering function of the kidney is the
   a. cortex
   b. medulla
   c. nephron
   d. pelvis

2. Considering the terms below, the one that does *not* indicate a renal function is
   a. filtration
   b. reabsorption
   c. dilution
   d. concentration

3. Acid-base balance is maintained by
   a. concentration
   b. hydrogen secretion
   c. elimination of bicarbonate
   d. retention of ammonia

4. The major constituent of urine is
   a. water
   b. potassium
   c. ammonia
   d. urea

5. The amount of reabsorption of water that takes place is dependent upon the level of
   a. ADH
   b. hydrogen
   c. bicarbonate
   d. renal threshold

Unit 1

6. In order to eliminate drugs from the body, the kidney uses the metabolic process of
   a. concentration
   b. reabsorption
   c. secretion
   d. dilution

7. The substance which is found in urine but is not a solute is
   a. urea
   b. bicarbonate
   c. creatinine
   d. bacteria

8. Of the urinary constituents below, the one whose concentration is regulated by aldosterone is
   a. urea
   b. sodium
   c. bilirubin
   d. creatinine

9. Cellular components are not filtered at the glomerulus because they are
   a. not present in the blood
   b. too large
   c. too small
   d. not a proper shape to fit in the tubules

10. Substances which are eliminated in the urine because of toxic effects include
    a. sodium
    b. bicarbonate
    c. bilirubin
    d. red cells

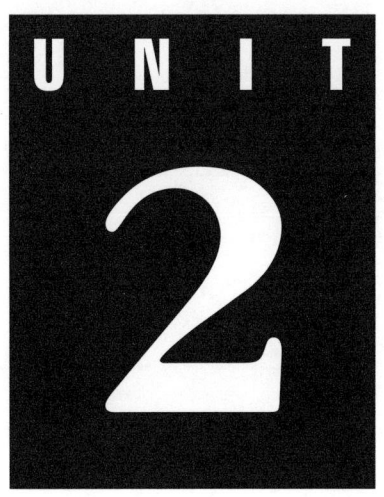

Quality Control and Safety in the Urinalysis Laboratory

LEARNING OBJECTIVES

After studying this unit, it is the responsibility of the student to know the following objectives:

- Define all terms in the glossary.
- State the purpose of quality control in the urinalysis laboratory.
- Outline the quality control necessary for chemical analysis of urines using reagent strips.
- Discuss the origins and use of urinalysis controls.
- Differentiate internal and external quality control.
- Outline Universal Precautions guidelines.
- Discuss safety practices in the urinalysis laboratory.

• Unit 2

GLOSSARY

biohazardous an agent that has the ability to cause infection in humans.

external quality control quality control procedures which compare the laboratory with others.

flammability the ability to ignite or catch fire.

internal quality control quality control procedures that focus on a single laboratory.

lyophilized freeze-dried.

quality assurance a comprehensive system for monitoring the accuracy of test results.

quality control a system for monitoring the accuracy of test results within the scope of the clinical laboratory.

Universal Precautions a set of guidelines developed to protect health care workers from exposure to infectious agents.

INTRODUCTION

Diagnostic testing is the major focus of the clinical laboratory. The primary topics of discussion in this urinalysis manual will be test procedures and their interpretations. While performing and interpreting each test procedure, the technician must incorporate additional knowledge and information that makes the test procedures as accurate as possible. Technicians must use safe practices to protect themselves, their co-workers, and patients. The information presented in this unit will emphasize **quality control** and safety as they apply to the laboratory setting.

QUALITY CONTROL IN THE URINALYSIS LABORATORY

A system of quality control in the laboratory is designed to provide patient test results that are accurate and acceptable for reporting to the patient and physician. Realizing that performing a test is only a portion of providing an accurate test result, the concept of quality control is better expressed in an expanded concept known as **quality assurance.**

QUALITY ASSURANCE

Quality assurance is an all inclusive system including not only the laboratory's role in test performance, but also the steps preceding and following laboratory testing. It is vital for each laboratory to have a comprehensive system of quality assurance. The focus of this section will be the quality control that takes place in the laboratory (internal) and includes test performance, although this is not meant to downplay the importance of the other aspects of quality assurance.

SPECIMEN COLLECTION AND HANDLING

Collection of a proper urine specimen precedes laboratory test performance. Urinalysis requires that the specimen be collected using appropriate methods, in a proper container, with correct preservatives, and properly stored to maintain its integrity. Specimen collection will be discussed in detail in Unit 3. Quality control steps for the collection of a proper specimen will also be addressed in that unit.

TEST PERFORMANCE

Each portion of urinalysis testing has quality control that parallels the procedures being performed. Chemical testing is done using a reagent strip. (Refer to Unit 5 for specific information.) In order to ascertain that these strips are providing correct chemical analyses, controls with known values are used in parallel with the patient tests.

Controls have two possible origins. The controls may be made in the laboratory by pooling or combining many samples. This pooled sample is tested numerous times by multiple individuals to determine the range of values that will

▪ Unit 2

be acceptable. Once this has been done, the control is used in parallel testing with patient specimens.

Due to the tedious task of pooling specimens and performing multiple determinations, most laboratories purchase control materials from a commercial source. These control materials are pooled and tested in much the same manner as the "in-house" preparations described above. Following the initial testing, the control material is **lyophilized** and packaged for distribution.

Each commercial control is accompanied by a package insert. The insert provides directions for reconstituting the vial of control to transform it to liquid form. These controls require the addition of a specified volume of distilled water. In addition, the expected values for each chemical component contained in the vial can be found on each insert. The value ranges provide an estimate of the results that should be obtained each time the control is used.

Most laboratories use two levels of controls. One control is a "normal" control and will produce values within the normal range. The second control is an "abnormal" control. The values for some or all of the chemical analyses will be out of range for this control. Each control is evaluated as a parallel test within a time frame designated by laboratory policy. This time frame may be as often as every batch of tests or as infrequently as once per work shift.

When using controls in parallel with testing, it is important to record and analyze the values obtained *each time the control is used*. When a control result is obtained, the analysis of these values should take place immediately. If any portion of the control is found to be outside of the acceptable range, the patient results must be considered invalid and may not be reported to the patient or the physician. If multiple controls are used, all parameters on each control must be acceptable before patient results can be reported. These criteria may vary by laboratory.

EXERCISE 7   USE OF LYOPHILIZED CONTROLS

Individually or in small groups, the students should examine package inserts from lyophilized controls that are provided by the instructor. While examining these inserts, the students should determine the following:

1. Is each control considered a "normal" or "abnormal" control?
2. What are the recommendations for reconstituting each control vial?
3. What are the storage requirements for the control vials before reconstitution and after reconstitution?
4. What are the recommendations for frequency of use for each control?
5. With input from the instructor, confer in a small group and determine how often each control would be used in a 500-bed hospital and in a small group practice of family practitioners. Share this information with the class.

If test values are found to be out of range on a control, an investigation must be performed to determine what caused the variation and a correction made. The entire set of tests (patients and controls) must then be repeated. Only if all parameters are acceptable on the repeat analysis can test results be considered valid.

Results for all control values must be permanently recorded. These records must include corrective actions for controls that were out of range. Recording systems should follow the protocol of the specific laboratory.

INSTRUMENT MAINTENANCE

All equipment necessary for performing urinalysis must be routinely monitored and maintained. This equipment will include items such as refrigerators, freezers, pipettes, centrifuges, microscopes, and refractometers. Records of these procedures are maintained in the standard format used in the laboratory. The records are necessary for licensing and accreditation purposes. Specific information on the necessary records may be obtained from the agencies that routinely visit laboratories for inspections (*e.g.,* College of American Pathologists [CAP] or Joint Commission on Accreditation of Healthcare Organizations [JCAHO]).

PROCEDURE MANUALS

As in all major areas of the laboratory, a procedure manual must be available in the urinalysis department. The manual should contain protocols and procedures for all of the tests which are performed. This manual must be routinely reviewed and updated. The National Committee for Clinical Laboratory Standards has published guidelines for the development of procedure manuals. These standards should be consulted before writing a procedure manual.

EXERCISE 8 — ANALYSIS OF URINE CONTROL VALUES

In small groups, consider the following situation:

A student was performing chemical analyses on patient urine. Two controls were routinely performed in parallel with each batch of ten patient urines. On the second batch of urines during the day shift, the student recorded that the bilirubin on the abnormal control was lower than acceptable.

1. Outline how this situation should be handled.
2. Role play the student and the supervisor and resolve this control problem.
3. Another group of peers should critique the role play.
4. Reverse groups and repeat the role plays.
5. Working independently, write a one-paragraph summary of the response to the supervisor.
6. Instructor should check the paragraphs.

EXTERNAL QUALITY CONTROL

The various control methods described above reflect the **internal quality control** of the institution. These internal controls consist of all forms of quality control which originate within the institution. The results of such programs are recorded, analyzed, and evaluated within the laboratory.

External quality control involves outside agencies. Each agency provides materials for analysis. The results of the analyses are then sent to the providing agency for review. The results are compared with those obtained by other laboratories which have analyzed the same samples. External quality control is provided by agencies such as the CAP.

SAFETY IN THE URINALYSIS LABORATORY

The safety of workers within the laboratory is a major concern. There are categories of hazards that need to be addressed to ensure this safety. The categories include biological, chemical, fire, radioactivity, mechanical, and electrical. The Occupational Safety and Health Administration (OSHA) is responsible for providing standards for safe environments for both patients and employees. They require the availability of written safety manuals and organized safety programs for employees within the workplace.

BIOLOGICAL HAZARDS

A primary focus of the safety within the laboratory is **biohazardous** materials. All body fluids and tissues for analysis are considered biological hazards. This includes urine. The Centers for Disease Control and Prevention published a set of safe practices called **Universal Precautions,** which are summarized in Table 2.1. This list of guidelines provides a basis for the protection of healthcare workers, their co-workers, and patients from biohazards. It is strongly recommended that laboratory workers follow these guidelines carefully.

These procedures help to prevent transmission of infectious agents such as hepatitis B virus (HBV) and the human immunodeficiency virus (HIV), the agent responsible for acquired immunodeficiency syndrome (AIDS).

Table 2.1. Universal Precautions.

Consider all patients' blood and body fluids to be biohazardous.
Always wash hands before and after contact with patients.
Wear gloves when handling blood, body fluids, tissue, or contaminated surfaces.
Wear gloves and waterproof aprons, masks, and goggles if splashing can occur or during wound sterilization, endoscopy, dialysis, or postmortem procedures.
Dispose of all needles in puncture-proof boxes, which must be accessible in all rooms.
Minimize need for mouth-to-mouth resuscitation by keeping mouthpieces readily available on crash carts and in all areas where this need is possible.
Clean blood and body fluid spills with a solution of bleach (10%) and water or with a hospital disinfectant.
Immediately report all needle sticks, accidental splashes, and contamination of wounds or body fluids.

EXERCISE 9 — HANDWASHING TECHNIQUES

Students should practice the following exercise and then use this format consistently throughout their laboratory exercises.

1. Turn on faucets and adjust water temperature using paper towels; this prevents contact with potentially contaminated faucets.
2. Wet the skin and apply the amount of soap indicated by the manufacturer of the soap.
3. Scrub hands vigorously in a circular motion for 3 minutes. Be careful not to touch any part of the sink.
4. Rinse and dry hands.
5. Turn off faucets with paper towel.

Barrier Protection

Barrier precautions are available and offer the laboratory worker protection from potential biohazards. These barrier precautions include gloves, goggles, face shields, laboratory coats, aprons, gowns, and shoe covers. It is not necessary to wear all of the available protection at all times; rather technicians should use their judgment with regard to the likelihood of the creation of aerosols, splashes, or skin contact. In addition, the use of laboratory coats and gowns that are fluid resistant is an additional protection for preventing clothing and skin exposure to biohazards.

The minimum protection to provide protection from biohazards is the consistent use of gloves, goggles, and clothing covers (*i.e.*, laboratory coats, gowns, or aprons). The use of other items is at the discretion of the technician. In addition, one should be prudent in the changing of gloves during testing procedures to be certain that contamination of inanimate objects or other individuals does not occur.

Biohazardous waste disposal must be done in a manner to render it no longer hazardous. Individual laboratories have established protocols for disposing of waste. The waste must be placed into containers properly labeled for biohazardous material (see Figure 2.1). The materials are then autoclaved and incinerated. The option of using a disposal service is exercised by many institutions.

Accidental spills or contaminated surfaces must be wiped clean in a manner to render possible infectious agents ineffective. Biohazardous spills need to be decontaminated with a germicide proven to kill infectious agents or a 10% sodium hypochlorite (bleach) solution. Daily cleaning of work surfaces with the same solutions will help to prevent accidental contamination.

CHEMICAL HAZARDS

Chemicals may be hazardous with exposure. Hazards include toxicity, flammability, explosiveness, skin irritations or burns, or a combination of these effects. Chemicals are provided with a labeling system developed by the National Fire

• Unit 2

E X E R C I S E   **10**   **BIOHAZARD PROTECTION**

Divide the class into groups and role play the following:

1. An instructor counseling a student who is leaving the laboratory after completing a batch of urines who failed to wash her hands at the end of the laboratory session.
2. A student who notices another student biting his fingernails in the laboratory.
3. A laboratory supervisor who notices a staff member eating in the cafeteria while wearing her outermost lab coat.
4. A phlebotomist who notes that a fellow worker has discarded used gloves in the trash can designated for paper.

E X E R C I S E   **11**   **REMOVAL OF SOILED GLOVES**

The removal of soiled gloves is done in a fashion to avoid contamination of the skin. The following steps will prevent contamination. Using a clean pair of gloves, practice this procedure until you are comfortable with the steps.

1. With the thumb and index finger of one hand, pull the top of the glove on the opposite hand so that it is removed by turning it inside out. Be careful *not* to touch the skin on the wrist area above the top of the glove.
2. Place that glove into the palm of the hand which is still gloved.
3. Using the hand with no glove, place the fingers of that hand inside the glove on the opposite hand.
4. Push the glove off so that it turns inside out and also covers the soiled glove which is being held in the palm.
5. What should be exposed is the inside of the second glove which was removed. Inside of that glove is the soiled surface and the entire glove which was removed first.
6. Discard these soiled gloves into a biohazardous waste container.

Quality Control and Safety in the Urinalysis Laboratory

EXERCISE 12 — SAFETY PROCEDURE

Divide the class into small groups. The instructor will provide sample safety manuals. Each group will:

1. Review a safety manual.
2. Write a safety procedure for protecting the technicians from biohazards in the urinalysis laboratory.
3. Share these procedures.

fig. 2.1. Biohazard label.

Protection Association (NFPA). Small quanitities of chemicals are used to perform tests in the urinalysis laboratory.

Employees need to be aware of the chemical hazards in their work environment. This is ensured by the OSHA requirement that material safety data sheets (MSDS) be provided for each chemical by manufacturers and suppliers. These sheets must be available on site for the chemicals utilized within the laboratory area.

Chemicals are provided with labels which identify the hazards inherent to each one. The National Fire Protection Association (NFPA) developed a labeling system in which all labels are a standard format (see Figure 2.2). Each label is divided into four color-coded sections. Each section provides information on a type of hazard: red designates **flammability,** blue indicates health hazards, yellow is the reactivity level, and white indicates special considerations. Within each of the four sections, a numerical assignment is made to indicate severity. These numbers are scaled 0 to 4, with 4 being the most hazardous. The label of each chemical container should be observed to determine potential hazards and handled in a manner to prevent accidents.

• Unit 2

EXERCISE 13 MSDS SHEETS

Instructors will divide the class into groups and provide each group with a MSDS sheet. The class will examine the sheet and determine the following:

1. Information provided on the sheet.
2. Interpretation of possible adverse effects of the chemical.

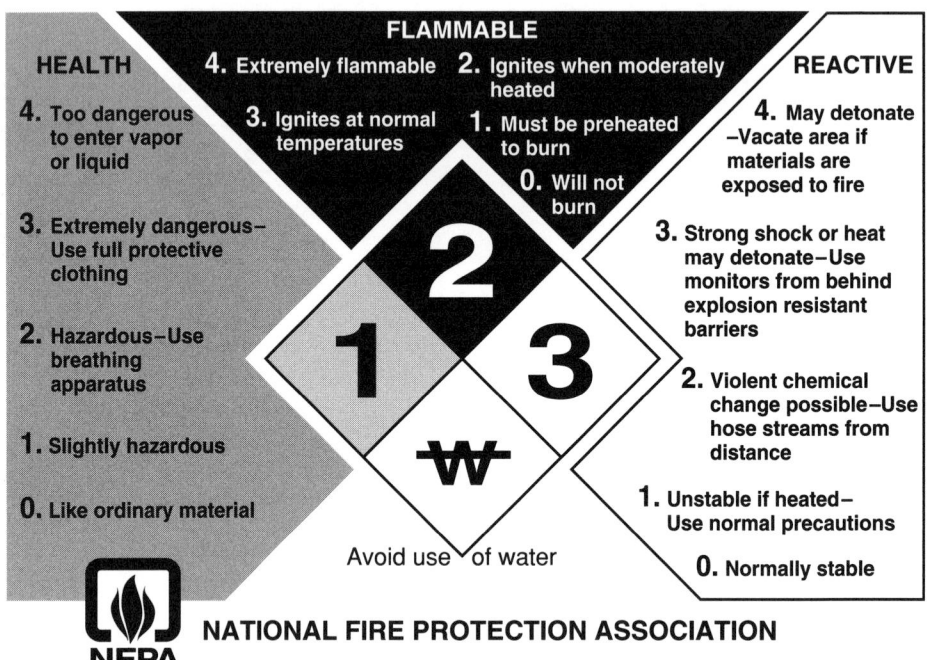

fig. 2.2. NFPA label. (Copyright © 1990, National Fire Protection Association, Quincy, MA 02269. This warning system is intended to be interpreted and applied only by properly trained individuals to identify fire, health, and reactivity hazards of chemicals. The user is referred to certain limited number of chemicals with recommended classifications in NFPA 49 and NFPA 325M, which would be used as a guideline only. Whether the chemicals are classified by NFPA or not, anyone using the 704 systems to classify chemicals does so at their own risk.)

Accidents can be further reduced by using fume hoods, carriers for caustic chemicals, gloves, goggles, aprons, and other protective coverings when handling chemicals. Appropriate storage of chemicals in specially ventilated cabinets is also necessary. As with biohazards, mouth pipetting is prohibited to reduce the possibility of injury by exposure to caustic chemicals.

Chemical spills should be properly removed with the use of a chemical spill kit. These kits should be available in areas of the laboratory where chemicals are

EXERCISE 14 NFPA LABELS

The instructor will divide the class into small groups and provide samples of NFPA labels. Each group will:

1. Examine the NFPA labels on a minimum of five different chemical containers.
2. Determine how the sections of the label distinguish hazards.
3. Research the NFPA labeling system with materials provided by the instructor.
4. Determine if their conclusions under #2 were correct.

EXERCISE 15 LOCATION OF SAFETY EQUIPMENT

Each student should explore a urinalysis or other laboratory.

1. Determine the location of all fire extinguishers.
2. Prepare a floor plan of the laboratory.
   a. Location of fire extinguishers (labeled with type).
   b. Flammable chemical cabinets.
   c. Fire blankets.
   d. Exits.
3. Develop a fire escape plan and include it on the map.

used. Disposal of chemicals should be according to the nature of the substance. Disposing of chemicals down drains or sewers is often not acceptable and it is sometimes necessary to use disposal companies.

ADDITIONAL HAZARDS

Hazards found in other areas of the laboratory are also applicable in urinalysis. Mechanical hazards are encountered when working with equipment such as centrifuges and automated reagent strip readers. Long hair should be tied back and loose clothing and jewelry secured or removed to prevent becoming entangled in moving parts.

Equipment and chemicals provide potential fire hazards. Fire extinguishers must be located throughout the laboratory. Technicians must distinguish the type of fire extinguishers (A, B, C) available and be experienced in the use of each. Fire escape plans should be posted and fire drills conducted periodically.

SUMMARY

Test performance is the main focus of the urinalysis laboratory. Whereas the focus remains on the methodologies and concurrent results, there are additional considerations. As discussed above, quality control helps to ascertain that the test results are accurate. Internal and external quality control are two broad systems used to monitor test methods. Quality control also includes the routine use of control materials in parallel testing, instrument maintenance, as well as proper specimen collection and recording methods. Quality control should remain an integral part of testing and record keeping.

Safety is also a vital component to the daily workings of the urinalysis laboratory. Safety must be consistently addressed to protect all of the persons working in the department. It is the responsibility of all employees to protect themselves as well as their co-workers. Use of barrier protections and eyeware and proper disposal of all materials are imperative for the safety of all exposed persons.

REVIEW QUESTIONS

1. Lyophilized controls are most often used in the urinalysis laboratory
   a. never more often than once daily
   b. at least once per hour
   c. with each batch of urines
   d. not at all
2. Normal and abnormal controls are both used in the urinalysis laboratory. On a batch of ten urines, the abnormal control was out of range for glucose. The technician should report patient results that are
   a. within the normal range only
   b. within the abnormal range only
   c. in all ranges
   d. none of the above
3. Quality control that takes place during the testing of urines is known as
   a. external
   b. maintenance
   c. internal
   d. permanent
4. A biological hazard is one that is
   a. caustic
   b. flammable
   c. infectious
   d. radioactive

5. Universal Precautions helps to
   a. protect health care workers from infectious disease ✓
   b. prevent fires
   c. avoid radioactive contamination
   d. dispose of chemical wastes
6. In the NFPA labeling system, a highly flammable liquid would have a 4 in the
   a. red quadrant ✓
   b. blue quadrant
   c. yellow quadrant
   d. white quadrant
7. A specially ventilated cabinet would be necessary to store
   a. radioactive materials
   b. biohazards
   c. fire extinguishers
   d. certain chemicals ✓
8. Mouth pipetting is permitted in the urinalysis laboratory
   a. at all times
   b. when pipetting water
   c. to measure control material
   d. at no time ✓
9. Safety in the workplace is the responsibility of the organization known as
   a. OSHA ✓
   b. NFPA
   c. MSDS
   d. CAP
10. The word lyophilized means
    a. liquid form
    b. biohazardous
    c. freeze dried ✓
    d. an aerosol

UNIT 3

Specimen Collection

LEARNING OBJECTIVES

After studying this unit, it is the responsibility of the student to know the following objectives:

- Discuss the importance of proper specimen collection.

- Describe containers appropriate for collection of specimens for routine urinalysis, timed collection, and microbiological analyses.

- Outline labeling procedures for urine specimens.

- Differentiate first morning specimen, random specimen, and pooled urine specimen.

- Describe a clean catch midstream urine specimen.

- List the four different preservatives and their uses.

GLOSSARY

clean catch a urine specimen usually collected in a sterile container, named clean catch since the glans penis and urethral meatus, in men and women respectively, are cleaned prior to collection.

diabetes mellitus a disease characterized by decreased carbohydrate metabolism due to decreased insulin, resulting in high blood and urine glucose levels.

diurnal occurring during the day.

fasting abstaining from food for a period of time.

first morning specimen the first specimen collected upon rising in the morning.

glucose tolerance test a test tracking the level of glucose in blood and urine, usually conducted over 2 to 4 hours.

midstream urine that excludes the first and last voided urine.

opaque impervious to the passage of light.

random specimen a specimen collected utilizing no particular method, container, or timing.

timed specimen a specimen collected either at a specified time or over an established time frame.

translucent slightly penetrable with light rays.

two-hour postprandial 2 hours after a meal.

Unit 3

INTRODUCTION

As with any laboratory analysis, the test procedure begins with collecting a proper specimen. The specimen must be collected by an acceptable method, in a container which will preserve its integrity, and consist of a volume sufficient for testing. If any of these items are not properly accounted for, the results of the urinalysis may be misleading or result in false-positive or false-negative results. This, in turn, could have grave consequences for the patient.

The collection of the urine specimen is most often done by the patient or health care professional other than the Medical Laboratory Technician. The technician, however, will frequently be responsible for determining procedures for specimen collection and will determine if the specimen received is appropriate for testing.

SPECIMEN CONTAINERS AND LABELING

The container appropriate for collection of a urine specimen for analysis depends on the tests being performed. The container to be used for routine urinalysis should be clean, dry, and composed of a material that is clear or **translucent.** All specimen containers must have an opening sufficient to accommodate the convenient collection of the specimen and be able to contain a minimum of 50 ml of urine. The container should have a lid which can be securely attached to prevent spillage of potentially biohazardous material while transporting. Disposable containers prevent accidental contamination and reduce the technician's exposure to biohazardous material. Specimens collected for microbiological culture must be collected into containers with sterile interiors.

Containers of appropriate volume must be provided for collection of 12- and 24-hour urines. These containers are light resistant and are most frequently made of brown **opaque** plastic with a leak-resistant cap. Containers for infant and pediatric patients are also available. See Figure 3.1 for samples of urine collection devices.

Labeling of all containers is vital. The label needs to be self-adhering and moisture resistant. The label should be securely attached to the container—*never* solely to a removable lid. It is acceptable for the label to be attached to the lid and the container. The label must be imprinted with patient identification as indicated by specific institutional guidelines. The minimum label requirements include name, identification number, room number, time, and date. Additional information may be specified by the institutional policies.

TYPES OF SPECIMENS

The easiest and most frequently collected urine sample is the **random specimen.** It is the most convenient for the patient to collect and provides a good screening for the individual's metabolic and renal systems. It is collected at any

Specimen Collection

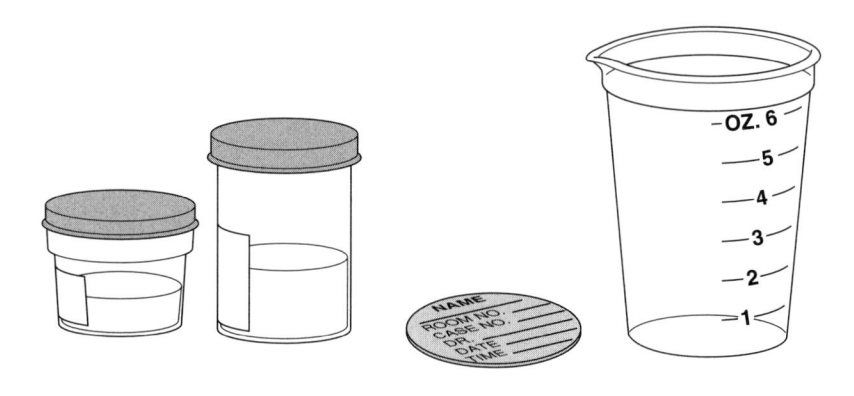

fig. 3.1. Urine collection containers.

EXERCISE 16 URINE CONTAINERS

Working in groups, the students will examine various urine specimen collection containers. They should:

1. Note any preservatives that have been added.
2. Determine whether the container is sterile.
3. Note whether it is designed for adults or infants.
4. Construct a table for future reference.

---

time and does not require any special instructions or preparations. This type of specimen is appropriate for routine urinalysis, as well as some analytes that do not require concentrated specimens or are not affected by **diurnal** variations.

The specimen of choice for clinicians is generally the **first morning specimen.** This specimen provides a concentrated sample of urine which contains a higher concentration of chemical constituents and microscopic elements. This sample can also serve as a baseline against which other samples can be measured and as a **fasting** specimen for the measurement of glucose. The patient is instructed to void before going to bed and to collect the first specimen upon rising in the morning.

Both the random and first morning specimens can be collected via the **midstream** method. This involves having the patient begin to void into the toilet or bedpan, thus discarding the initial urine. The patient then collects the "midstream" into an appropriate container. Once an adequate amount is collected, the remaining urine is directed into the toilet or bedpan and discarded. A midstream specimen is preferred for microbiological studies since it is less likely to be contaminated with organisms surrounding the genitalia. A variation of this method is the **clean catch** midstream specimen. A midstream clean catch specimen is preferable for microbiological studies. This method involves cleaning the genitalia with a mild antiseptic prior to collecting the midstream specimen. This, in turn, will further reduce the likelihood of bacterial contamination. Patients must be instructed regarding how to properly collect a midstream clean catch urine. The instructions should be given clearly and concisely, both verbal and written. Finally, when a patient's primary or first language is not English, every attempt should be made to give the instructions in the patient's native language.

The **timed specimen** may be either a specimen collected at a specified time or over a period of time. Fasting specimens are those collected after a period of time, at least 8 hours, in which the patient has not consumed food or drink, although water may be permissible. At the beginning of the fast, the patient should void and discard this urine.

The **two-hour postprandial** specimen is a very common timed specimen. The patient voids and discards this urine, then consumes a normal meal. After 2 hours, a specimen is collected which is generally analyzed for urinary glucose. The 2-hour postprandial is a good screening test for **diabetes mellitus.** Another screening test for the presence of diabetes is the **glucose tolerance test.** After the patient has fasted for at least 12 hours, urine and blood are collected to establish a baseline glucose level. Following this, the patient will ingest a fixed amount of glucose, usually 100 grams in a liquid drink. Then, blood and urine are collected at predetermined timed intervals, initially every half hour, then every hour for up to 3 to 5 hours. The levels of glucose in the blood and urine are monitored, which in turn help in the diagnosis of diabetes mellitus.

Another type of timed urine specimen is a pooled urine specimen, which is the total urine produced and collected over a period of time. The time period is most often either 12 or 24 hours. This type of specimen is utilized for quantitative assays on urinary analytes such as casts and creatinine. The pooling of the specimen counteracts the effects of diurnal variation, hydration, exercise, and body metabolism on the results obtained from the analysis.

Similar to the midstream urine collections, the timed specimen requires specific procedures and instructions. These procedures and instructions must be explained to the patient or health care worker who will be collecting the specimen.

EXERCISE 17 CLEAN CATCH MIDSTREAM PROCEDURE

Working in pairs, students will:

1. Write a procedure for collection of a clean catch midstream urine collection.
2. Role play giving these instructions to a "patient."
3. Be observed and critiqued by the instructor.

Specimen Collection

PRESERVATIVES

Ideally, urine should be analyzed as soon as possible after collection but no later than 2 hours after collection. This eliminates the need for any type of preservation of the specimen. The most common form of preservation is refrigeration. This allows for a period of 4 hours to elapse before the specimen is no longer acceptable for analysis. A disadvantage of refrigeration is that amorphous urates or amorphous phosphates could precipitate, which could interfere with testing.

There are several chemical substances that are available to preserve urine specimens. Each has advantages and disadvantages regarding their effect on the various constituents of urine (see Table 3.1).

Additionally, various chemical preservatives have different applications for the various types of specimens collected (see Table 3.2). Finally, when using any type of chemical preservative, directions must be followed carefully and warnings must be heeded.

EXERCISE 18 — URINE SPECIMENS

Working individually, each student will construct a reference table for the various types of urine specimens. The table should include:

1. The name of the specimen.
2. Whether the specimen is a timed specimen.
3. What the specimen is used for.
4. Special patient preparation requirements (if any).

Table 3.1. Common Preservatives and Their Effect on Various Urine Analytes.

Preservative	Action	Comments
Refrigeration	Inhibits bacterial growth; does not interfere with chemical tests; precipitates amorphous phosphates and urates	Most common
Boric acid	Stabilizes pH around 6; maintains bacteria and will not interfere with routine urinalysis	Good for transporting culture specimens; provided in tablet form for ease of use
Formaldehyde	Preserves sediment constituents; interferes with copper reduction tests for glucose	May precipitate protein
Sodium fluoride	Inhibits glycolysis	Interferes with glucose, blood, and leukocyte reagent strip tests

Table 3.2. Various Urine Specimens; Their Applications and Preservatives.

Specimen	Use	Preservative
Random	Routine screening	None or refrigeration if not examined within 2 hours
First Morning	Routine screening Glucose monitoring Fasting	None or refrigeration if not examined within 2 hours
2-Hour Postprandial	Glucose monitoring	None or refrigeration if not examined within 2 hours
Glucose Tolerance Test	Glucose monitoring	None or refrigeration if not examined within 2 hours
12- or 24-Hour Collection	Quantitative analyses	Refrigeration plus boric acid or formaldehyde if sediment is of primary importance
Midstream Clean Catch Collection	Routine but especially microbiological studies	Refrigeration plus boric acid, especially if specimen is to be transported

EXERCISE 19 URINE PRESERVATIVES

Each student will construct a table about preservatives that:

1. Names the various preservatives.
2. Lists the effect of each on urine constituents.
3. Lists the applications for various urine specimens.

(Hint: See Tables 3.1 and 3.2.)

This may be combined with EXERCISE 18—URINE SPECIMENS.

SUMMARY

This unit demonstrates the importance of a properly collected urine specimen. Proper collection involves the type of container, the collection method, and the preservative. The collection method will vary according to the type of specimen required. Without a properly collected specimen, test results may be questionable. Subsequent chapters will discuss the analysis of urine specimens.

REVIEW QUESTIONS

1. A timed collection is a specimen which is collected
   a. after a period of fasting
   b. after a specified period of time
   c. excluding the first and last urine
   d. first thing in the morning

2. The preservative which inhibits glycolysis is
   a. boric acid
   b. calcium
   c. formaldehyde
   d. sodium fluoride

3. A urine collected after the initially voided urine is discarded is a
   a. fasting specimen
   b. random specimen
   c. timed specimen
   d. midstream specimen

4. A urine which is collected after no food or drink has been consumed for at least 8 hours is a
   a. fasting specimen
   b. random specimen
   c. timed specimen
   d. midstream specimen

5. A 2-hour postprandial is most often used for
   a. cholesterol screening
   b. glucose monitoring
   c. microbiological studies
   d. quantifying cellular components

6. Specimens for microbiological culture are collected into containers that
   a. have a preservative
   b. can contain 1000 ml
   c. have sterile interiors
   d. are not disposable

7. The type of specimen which does *not* usually require special patient instructions is the
   a. fasting specimen
   b. random specimen
   c. timed specimen
   d. midstream clean catch specimen

- Unit 3

8. A urine sample is transported to the laboratory. From the descriptions listed below, choose the statement which indicates an error in labeling.
   a. only the lid is labeled
   b. the label is self-adhering
   c. patient's name and identification number are on the label
   d. the label is hand-written

9. A midstream urine is collected by
   a. collecting all urine into the container
   b. collecting some urine, discarding the next small amount, collecting the last portion of the specimen into a separate container
   c. discarding some urine, collecting a sufficient amount for testing, discarding the rest of the urine
   d. collecting all urine into a container and discarding a portion into the toilet or bedpan

10. Pooled urine is prepared by
    a. combining urine from many patients
    b. collecting all urine for a designated time period from one patient
    c. mixing urine from one patient for several days
    d. catching *portions* of many samples from one patient for 12 hours

UNIT 4

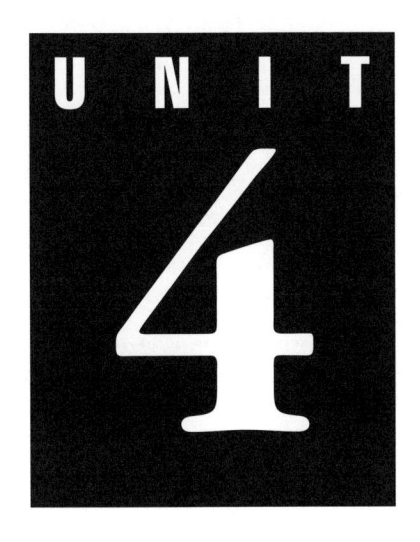

Physical Examination of Urine

LEARNING OBJECTIVES

After studying this unit, it is the responsibility of the student to know the following objectives:

- Define the terms that are used to describe normal urine.

- Discuss the constituents that give urine its color, both normal and abnormal.

- Define specific gravity and discuss how it is measured.

- Determine when and how to perform corrections to specific gravity due to both temperature and high concentrations of glucose and protein.

- Describe and discuss the appearance of amorphous urates and amorphous phosphates in urine.

- List the causes and discuss the significance of abnormalities in urine.

- Discuss the reasons for abnormally high and low specific gravity urine.

- Define terms listed in the glossary.

GLOSSARY

amorphous phosphates crystals that precipitate in alkaline urine, considered normal; give urine a white hue.

amorphous urates crystals that precipitate in acidic urine, considered normal; give urine a pink hue.

bilirubin breakdown product of hemoglobin; gives urine a dark yellow or amber color.

diabetes insipidus a condition characterized by polyuria (increased urine output) resulting from the increased secretion of antidiuretic hormone (ADH) or the inability of the kidneys to respond to ADH.

glomerulonephritis an inflammation of the glomerulus of the kidney; symptoms include decreased urine production and the presence of protein and blood in the urine.

hemoglobin a substance found in red blood cells that transports oxygen to muscles and tissues and transports carbon dioxide to the lungs.

hypersthenuria urine with an abnormally high specific gravity.

hyposthenuria urine with an abnormally low specific gravity.

maple syrup urine disease a disease in which the patient cannot metabolize certain amino acids, recognized by the maple syrup odor present in the urine.

pyelogram an x-ray picture of the kidneys and ureters after the injection of a dye.

pyelonephritis bacterial infection of the kidney.

turbid a nontransparent appearance, usually with particulate matter such as bacteria or precipitates.

urochrome a pigment that gives urine its characteristic color.

Physical Examination of Urine

INTRODUCTION

As mentioned in Unit 1, historically the examination of urine was purely a physical examination. The ancient physicians examined the urine's color, odor, taste, and appearance, including turbidity and presence of foam. Today, while the taste and foam are no longer analyzed, the remaining physical characteristics, as well as specific gravity, are examined.

COLOR

The color of normal urine, caused by a pigment called **urochrome,** can be described along a continuum from pale yellow to amber (see Table 4.1). Generally speaking, the color of urine corresponds to the concentration of the liquid. Pale yellow or straw-colored urine will have a low concentration, whereas dark yellow or amber urine will have a higher concentration.

An abnormal color may be an indication of a pathologic condition and require further investigation. One of the more commonly encountered abnormal colors seen during routine urinalysis is pink or red. Often this is caused by the presence of red blood cells and/or **hemoglobin** which is secondary to a renal or urinary tract problem. Conversely, a pink or red urine may be normal in situations such as when a specimen is contaminated with menstrual blood or when individuals have eaten beets.

Another color that deserves mention is dark yellow or amber. Often this is a normal color in a highly concentrated urine and may be a result of strenuous exercise and/or dehydration. However, this color may also be associated with the presence of **bilirubin.** The presence of bilirubin, a metabolic product of hemoglobin, may be indicative of a hepatic disorder including hepatitis B. This possible scenario stresses the importance of always using Universal Precautions when working with urine as well as other body fluids. (See Table 4.2 for further examples of abnormal urine coloration.)

Table 4.1. The Color Range of Normal Urine.

Pale yellow*—Light yellow—Yellow—Dark yellow—Amber

*Straw is another term used for pale yellow.

Table 4.2. Abnormal Urine Colors.

Color	Possible Indications
Colorless	May be normal. May be an indication of kidneys lacking the ability to concentrate urine. Possibly an indication of diabetes insipidus.
Red/Pink	May be normal following the ingestion of beets or menstrual contamination. May be an indication of renal disease such glomerulonephritis, bladder infection or kidney stones with blood or hemoglobin (occasionally myoglobin) giving urine the red color.
Dark Yellow/Amber	May be normal, concentrated urine when associated with strenuous exercise or dehydration. May be indicative of hepatic disease with bilirubin causing the urine coloration.
Brown/Black	May be due to the presence of denatured hemoglobin. May also be seen in patients with alkaptonuria, a metabolic disorder resulting in homogentisic acid being excreted. The urine is normal in color initially but turns black when alkalinated.

■ Unit 4

| E X E R C I S E | 20 | URINE COLLECTION |

The instructor should:

1. Have each student in the laboratory collect a sample of their own urine.
2. Instruct each student to observe and record the color of their urine.
3. Designate a recorder to record the colors on a blackboard.
4. Lead a discussion of the significance of the colors observed.

APPEARANCE

The appearance of urine is generally described as clear, slightly cloudy or hazy, cloudy, or **turbid.** There are no industry-wide standards dictating specificities for appearance, but there should be consistency within each laboratory.

The appearance of urine should not be determined unless the urine is in a clear, preferably colorless, container. This may necessitate transferring some urine from its original container into one that fits this description. Normal, freshly voided urine is usually clear in appearance. Upon standing, normal acidic urine may become cloudy or turbid. This is due to the normal precipitation of **amorphous urates,** which will give the urine a pink hue. If the pH is basic or alkaline, white **amorphous phosphates** may precipitate. Again, this is a normal occurrence. Normal urine may be slightly cloudy upon voiding due to mucus or epithelial cells, especially in women.

Bacteria and white or red blood cells can give urine a cloudy appearance. The extent of the turbidity will vary with the amount of constituent present. The presence of bacteria or blood cells can be confirmed by chemical and/or microscopic analysis.

SPECIFIC GRAVITY

As previously discussed in Unit 1, a very important function of the kidney is the reabsorption of water and the excretion of waste products. Whenever water is selectively removed from a solution, in this case the glomerular filtrate, the solution becomes more concentrated. A way to monitor whether the kidney is performing this very important function is by measuring the specific gravity of the urine. Specific gravity is a ratio or comparison of the weight or density of a solution, such as urine, to an equal amount of distilled water which has a specific gravity of 1.000.

Initially, the glomerular filtrate has a specific gravity of 1.010. Normally, random urine collected from a healthy population will have a range of 1.015 to 1.025, although the range can be as wide as 1.001 to 1.035 depending on the state of hydration of the individual. Consistently low urine specific gravity (<1.010),

Physical Examination of Urine

EXERCISE 21 — URINE APPEARANCE

Using the urine collected for EXERCISE 20—URINE COLLECTION, the instructor should:

1. Instruct the students to observe and record the appearance of their urine.
2. Designate a recorder to record the appearances on a blackboard.
3. Lead a discussion of the significance of the various appearances observed.

known as **hyposthenuria,** may be an indication that the kidneys have lost the ability to concentrate urine. This may have grave consequences. Certain disease conditions directly affecting the kidney that may result in hyposthenuria are **pyelonephritis** and **glomerulonephritis. Diabetes insipidus,** while not a disease of the kidney, may also result in urine with a low specific gravity.

High specific gravity or **hypersthenuria** may result from conditions that cause dehydration in the patient such as vomiting, diarrhea, or strenuous exercise. Extremely high specific gravity, *i.e.*, above 1.035, is often associated with patients who have recently undergone procedures that required the use of radiographic contrast media, such as an intravenous **pyelogram** or other diagnostic imaging procedures.

There are several ways to measure the specific gravity of urine—by urinometer, refractometer, and reagent strips. A urinometer is a device that will measure specific gravity of urine via a specially designed weighted float which is suspended in urine (see Fig 4.1). There are several disadvantages to using a urinometer. First, it requires a large volume of urine, about 10 to 15 ml. Whereas this may not be a problem for most people, this volume is impractical for pediatric and neonatal patients as well as patients who may be dehydrated. Also, urinometers are calibrated to be used at a fixed temperature. This is usually around 20° C and will be stated on the urinometer. If the room temperature or specimen deviates from this, the reading must be corrected. Therefore, for every 3° the temperature is below the calibration temperature 0.001 must be subtracted from the reading and for every 3° the temperature is above the calibration temperature 0.001 must be added to the reading. Another correction involves subtracting 0.003 for each gram per deciliter (gm/dl) of urine protein and 0.004 for each gm/dl of urine glucose from the specific gravity reading present in urine.

A refractometer is probably the most common way that specific gravity is measured (see Figures 4.2 and 4.3). Refractometers measure the refractive index, which is a comparison of the speed of light in air with the speed of light in a solution. The principle is that light bends as it enters a solution because its speed is decreased. The more concentrated the solution (the higher the specific gravity), the more the light bends, meaning that it has a higher refractive index. Within the refractometer is a scale that converts the refractive index into specific gravity. The great advantage of the refractometer is that it requires only one or

• Unit 4

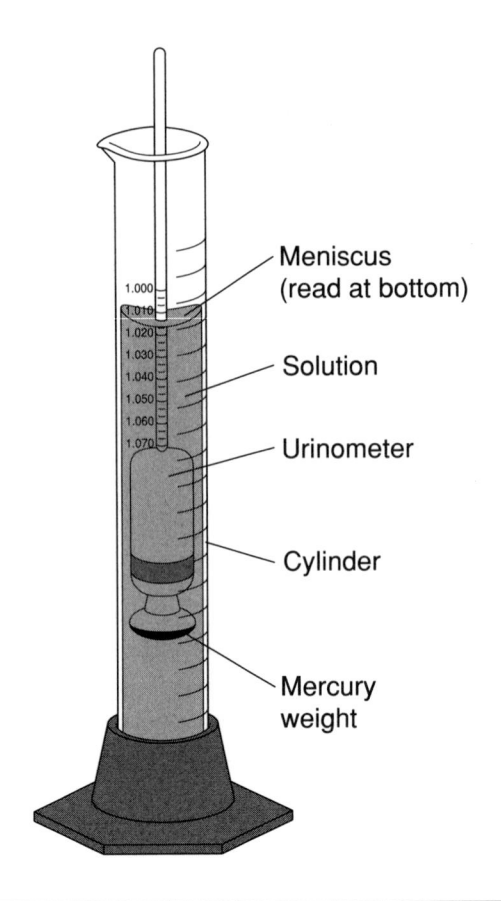

fig. 4.1. Urinometer; specific gravity is read off the graduated scale on the stem of the urinometer.

E X A M P L E

The specific gravity using a urinometer calibrated at 20° C is 1.025. The room temperature is 17° C and there is 1 gm/dl of protein present. What is the corrected specific gravity?

Solution: $1.025 - 0.001^* - 0.003^\dagger = 1.021$

*Correction for temperature.
†Correction for protein.

E X E R C I S E **22** **CALCULATING SPECIFIC GRAVITY**

Each student should solve the following problem:

The specific gravity using a urinometer calibrated at 20° C is 1.028. The room temperature is 23° C and there are 2 gm/dl of glucose present. What is the corrected specific gravity?

two drops of urine, thus making it ideal for situations where only a small amount of urine is available. It does not require correction for temperature but does require protein and glucose correction similar to the urinometer corrections.

A third common way to measure specific gravity is by using reagent strips. This is a chemical method and is not as sensitive as the two physical methods, in that the reagent strips provide readings in 0.005 increments. A urine pH of 6.5 or greater may interfere with the reaction; therefore, 0.005 should be added to specific gravity readings when the pH is in this range. Elevated protein levels may also cause increases in the readings.

ODOR

One aspect of urinalysis that is no longer routinely reported is odor. It is seldom clinically significant and is never the sole means for detecting any type of infection or disorder. Normal urine will have an aromatic odor which will acquire an

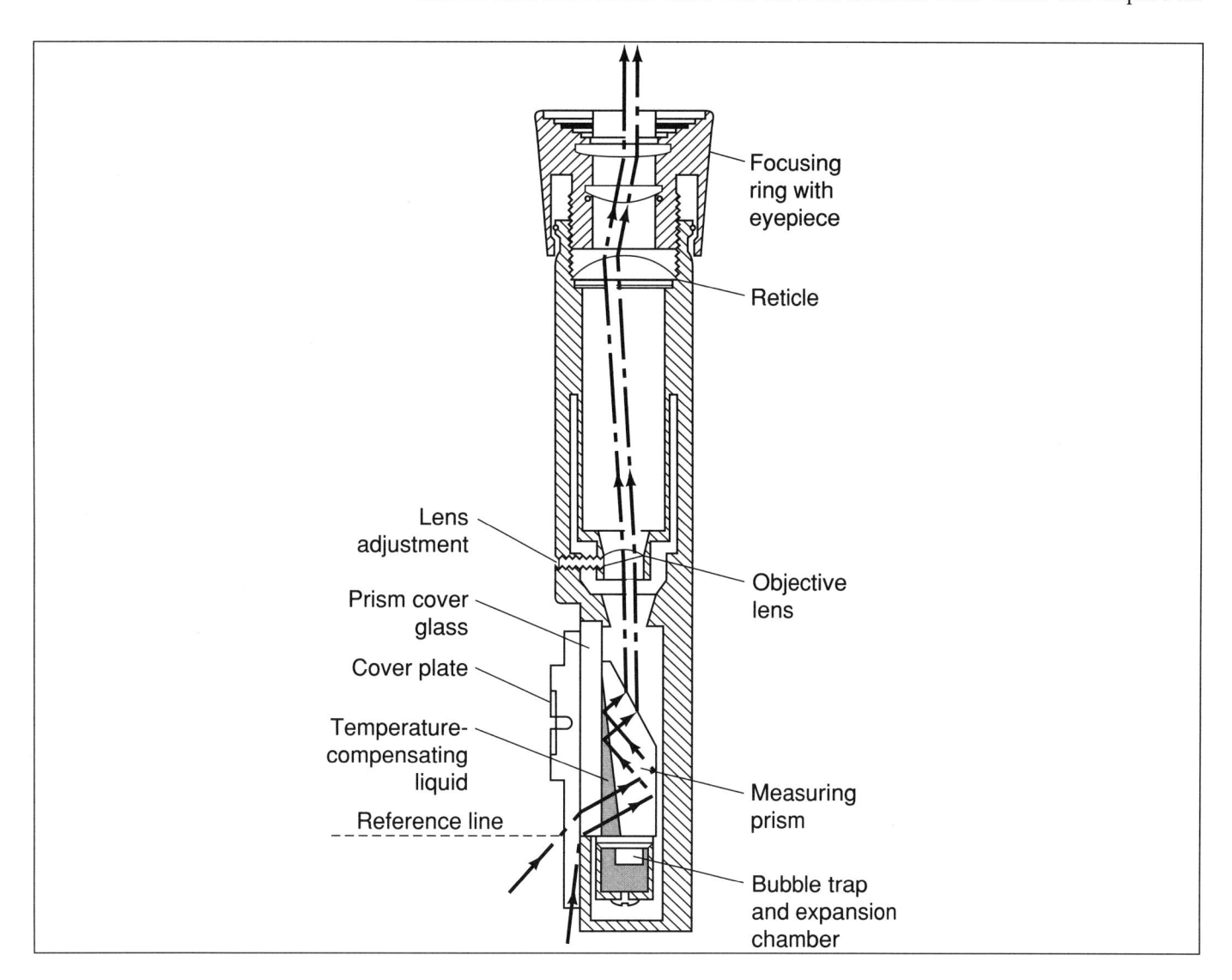

fig. 4.2. Refractometer; a schematic representation. (Courtesy of Leica, Inc. Buffalo, NY.)

■ Unit 4

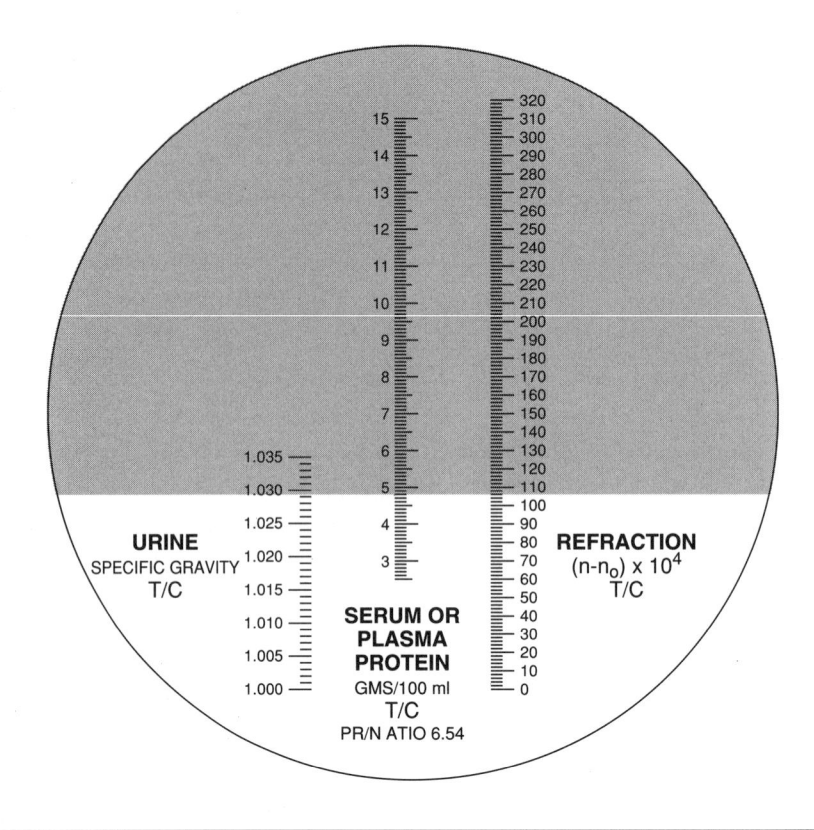

fig. 4.3. Refractometer scale as it would appear in the refractometer. (Courtesy of Leica, Inc. Buffalo, NY.)

EXERCISE 23 COMPARING THE URINOMETER AND REFRACTOMETER

Working in small groups, the students should do the following:

1. Using the urinometer, determine the specific gravity of five urines collected for EXERCISE 20—URINE COLLECTION.
2. Using the refractometer, determine the specific gravity of the same five urines.
3. Make a chart and compare the results.
4. Discuss why the results are or are not the same.

ammonia odor upon standing due to the breakdown of urea. However, there are times when detecting the odor may be helpful in the early detection of a disease such as **maple syrup urine disease,** an inherited metabolic disorder. Additionally, after the ingestion of certain food, especially asparagus, urine may have a distinctive odor.

SUMMARY

The physical examination of urine is a critical component of the urinalysis. The color, appearance, and specific gravity each reflect an aspect of the health status of the kidneys. It is important for the technician to distinguish between normal and possible pathological physical characteristics. The odor, as well as taste and appearance of foam, while once playing a critical role, contribute only a minor role in the overall urinalysis today.

REVIEW QUESTIONS

1. The presence of this compound may be indicative of a hepatic disorder
   a. bilirubin
   b. hemoglobin
   c. ammonia
   d. intact red blood cells
2. Which of the following is the pigment that gives urine its characteristic color?
   a. hemoglobin
   b. biliverdin
   c. homogentisic acid
   d. urochrome
3. These crystals give urine a pink tint
   a. amorphous phosphates
   b. cholesterol
   c. amorphous urates
   d. tyrosine
4. Hyposthenuria is urine with
   a. a consistently low specific gravity
   b. a consistently high specific gravity
   c. a normal specific gravity
   d. a specific gravity of 1.000
5. Compared to a urinometer, a refractometer
   a. uses the same amount of urine
   b. does require a temperature correction
   c. uses less urine
   d. can only determine specific gravity in increments of 0.005
6. This color of urine may be indicative of hepatic disease
   a. red
   b. green
   c. straw
   d. amber

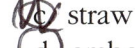

Unit 4

7. Amorphous phosphates may cause the urine to have the following color
   a. red
   (b.) white
   c. straw
   (d.) amber
8. A disadvantage of the urinometer is
   a. it requires a small amount of urine
   (b.) it requires a large amount of urine
   c. it cannot be used if the room temperature is not 20° C
   d. it cannot be used it there is high urine glucose
9. A urinometer is calibrated at 20° C. A patient's urine has a reading of 1.022 with 2 gm/dl of urine protein present. The room temperature is 23° C. What result should be reported?
   a. 1.015
   (b.) 1.017
   c. 1.020
   d. 1.022
10. A urinometer is calibrated at 22° C. A patient's urine has a reading of 1.022 with 1 gm/dl of urine glucose present. The room temperature is 22° C. What result should be reported?
    a. 1.017
    (b.) 1.018
    c. 1.019
    d. 1.020

FURTHER ACTIVITIES

In small groups, contact local hospitals and inquire how they measure specific gravity and what backup procedure is used. Summarize the findings in a short report to be given to the instructor. Give an oral report to the class.

UNIT 5

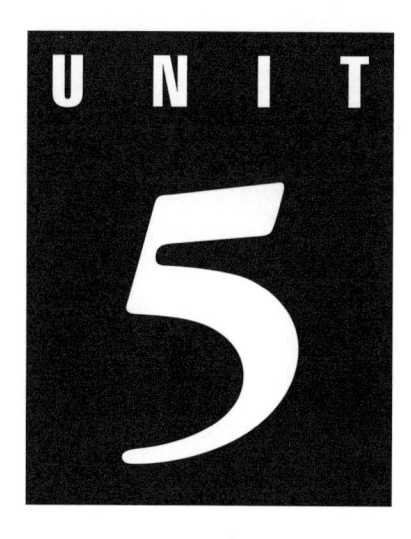

Chemical Examination of Urine

LEARNING OBJECTIVES

After studying this unit, it is the responsibility of the student to know the following objectives:

- Discuss the proper use of and key reactants in chemical reagent strips.

- List the causes of false-positive and false-negative results for each of the analytes when using chemical reagent strips.

- Discuss appropriate use and principles of supplementary tests.

- State the significance of a positive reaction in each chemical test.

- Describe the principle of operation for automated chemical reagent strip readers.

- Define terms listed in the glossary.

GLOSSARY

calculi (singular, calculus) commonly referred to as a stone, a deposit made of mineral salts.

carbohydrate chemical substance made of hydrogen, oxygen, and carbon; primary source of energy.

chromagen a color indicator.

desiccant a substance to withdraw moisture.

enzyme a protein that may catalyze a chemical change.

galactosemia the presence of galactose in the blood; an inborn error of metabolism resulting in the inability to convert galactose to glucose.

galactosuria galactose in the urine.

glomerulonephritis an inflammation of the glomerulus of the kidney; symptoms include decreased urine production and the presence of protein and blood in the urine.

glucosuria an abnormal amount of glucose in the urine.

glycosuria synonymous with glucosuria.

granulated leukocyte leukocytes that contain granules in their cytoplasm; these include neutrophils, basophils, and eosinophils; also known as a granulocyte.

hematuria the appearance of blood in the urine.

hemoglobin a substance found in red blood cells that transports oxygen to muscles and tissues and transports carbon dioxide to the lungs.

hemoglobinuria blood in the urine, but not the presence of intact red blood cells.

jaundice a condition resulting from increased bilirubin in the blood and characterized by a yellowing of the skin and sclera (the white part of the eyes).

multiple myeloma a tumor disease of the bone, characterized by increased protein production.

myoglobin a globulin found in muscle tissue.

orthostatic proteinuria a protein in the urine that is a result of a shift in postural position.

proteinuria abnormal amount of protein in the urine.

INTRODUCTION

One of the most common and simple diagnostic laboratory tests is the chemical analysis of urine. This is usually performed following the physical examination of urine. Although a simple test, it reveals a great deal of information about various systems and organs of the body, most notably the renal and urogenital systems. This unit will describe and discuss the various chemical tests that are routinely performed on urine as well as some of the most common confirmatory tests.

REAGENT STRIPS

The primary tool used in the chemical analysis of urine is the reagent strip, commonly referred to as the dipstick. The reagent strip is an inert plastic strip with several small pads attached. Each pad is designed to perform a different chemical analysis by virtue of the reagents that are impregnated in the pad. The reagents in each pad will produce a color reaction after coming into contact with a particular substance in the urine. The resulting color is compared to a chart provided on the reagent bottle to determine the result of the test. Depending on the test, the results may be reported as negative through 3+ or 4+ (bilirubin and blood), in concentrations such as mg/dl (protein, glucose, ketone, and urobilinogen) or in a conventional manner (pH and specific gravity).

Reagent strips may be purchased with single or multiple tests available. (See Table 5.1 for a summary of the reagent strips available and the tests performed by each. Strips commonly are purchased in an opaque bottle that is used for storage. The bottle contains a **desiccant** to decrease moisture in the bottle which may interfere when testing is performed. The strips must not be exposed to temperatures greater than 30° C, and it is recommended that they be stored at room temperature. Only the number of strips to be used at a given time should be removed from the bottle. The bottle should be tightly closed at all times. As with any reagent, the manufacturer's instructions should be closely followed. (See Table 5.2 for a summary of the proper way to use a reagent strip.)

Table 5.1. Common Chemistry Reagent Strips.

	pH	Specific Gravity	Protein	Glucose	Ketones	Blood	Nitrite	Bilirubin	Urobilinogen	Leukocyte Esterase
Ames Multistix	X		X	X	X	X		X	X	
Ames N-Multistix	X		X	X	X	X	X	X	X	
Ames Multistix 10	X	X	X	X	X	X	X	X	X	X
Chemstrip 10SG	X	X	X	X	X	X	X	X	X	X
Chemstrip 9	X		X	X	X	X	X	X	X	X
Chemstrip 8	X		X	X	X	X		X	X	X
Chemstrip 7	X		X	X	X	X		X		X

Table 5.2. Proper Use of Reagent Strip.

1. Obtain a fresh urine specimen. It should be collected in a clean dry container. If refrigerated, it should be allowed to return to room temperature.
2. Remove a single strip from the bottle. Be sure to replace the cap tightly.
3. Immerse the strip completely in the urine and remove promptly. While removing the strip from the urine, run the edge along the rim of the urine container to remove excess urine.
4. Hold the strip horizontally against the reaction chart and read the various reactions at the appropriate times as indicated by the manufacturer.

EXERCISE 24 CHEMICAL REAGENT STRIPS

Working in small groups with sample reagent strips supplied by the instructor:

1. Examine the reagent strip and container and note which tests can be done.
2. Note the ranges and sensitivity of the various tests.
3. On the blackboard, overhead, etc., construct a table with the notes from each group of students.

pH

One of the functions of the kidneys is to regulate the acid-base balance in the blood. This is done by regulating the amount of hydrogen ion secreted in the urine. Urinary pH is a measure of the hydrogen ion concentration in the urine. Normal, freshly voided urine has a pH of 5.0 to 6.0, although pH ranging from 4.5 to 8.0 may be normal. A urine pH below 4.5 or above 8.0 is probably an indication of an improperly collected or stored sample and may not be suitable for further testing. A new specimen should be requested in a clean container.

The test method for determining the pH on a reagent strip is based on the reaction of color indicators with hydrogen ions in the urine. There are two indicators in the reagent pad, bromthymol blue and methyl red. Methyl red ranges in color from red to yellow in pH 4.4 to 6.2 and bromthymol blue ranges from yellow to blue in pH 6.0 to 7.6.

Knowledge of the urinary pH is important in identifying crystals, such as uric acid, that may be found in urine. An acidic urine may be associated with clinical conditions such as starvation, diabetes mellitus, and respiratory disease, whereas an alkaline urine may be seen with prolonged vomiting or in association with a vegetarian diet. Urinary pH is also important in attempting to control the formation of kidney stones or **calculi.** Calculi form in alkaline urine; therefore, if an individual is prone to kidney stone formation it is very helpful to maintain an acidic urine.

Fortunately, there are not significant substances that interfere with the pH testing on the reagent strip. However, caution must be exercised when performing the test since "runover" from adjacent acidic reagent pads may produce a falsely low pH reading.

Chemical Examination of Urine

PROTEIN

The determination of protein in urine may be the single most important factor in screening for renal disease. The presence of protein in urine is termed **proteinuria** and serves as an early warning sign of renal disease. Normal urine contains a small amount of protein, mostly albumin. Another normal protein found in the urine is Tamm-Horsfall protein produced in the tubules and collecting ducts of the nephron. However, this small quantity, usually less than 10 mg/dl, is not detected in routine protein determination using the reagent strip.

Most protein is not filtered across the glomerular membrane of the nephrons. The majority of filtered protein is reabsorbed in the tubules. However, if there is any damage to the glomerular membrane, there will be an increase in the amount of protein in the urine. There are several conditions that can cause damage to the glomerular membrane, including acute **glomerulonephritis**, toxins, immunologic reactions, and infections.

Other sources of protein in the urine may be prerenal, from renal tubular damage, or originating in the lower urinary tract. A prerenal condition that results in increased protein production is **multiple myeloma.** This condition results in increased production of low molecular weight proteins that are filtered across the glomerular membrane and exceed the reabsorption capacity of the tubules. Thus it can be detected in the urine.

Similarly, if the tubules are damaged and cannot reabsorb protein, it will pass into the urine. Lastly, an infection in the lower urinary tract, including the bladder, will result in urinary protein.

A nonpathological condition of proteinuria worth mentioning is **orthostatic proteinuria**, sometimes called postural proteinuria. This condition results in urinary protein appearing as a result of the patient changing postural position from lying down to sitting or standing. (See Table 5.3 for a procedure to screen for orthostatic proteinuria.)

Using the reagent strips, detection of urinary protein is based on a test referred to as "Protein Error of Indicators." At a constant pH of 3.0, the presence of protein will cause a color indicator to change. The amount of color change is directly proportional to the amount of protein in the urine. A buffer in the reagent pad maintains the pH at 3.0. This is why care must be taken to avoid allowing excess fluid to remain on the reagent strip. The acidic condition of the protein pad could cause a false low reading on the adjacent pH pad.

The principal protein detected in the reagent strip test is albumin. This is a relatively low molecular weight protein that is filtered across the glomerular membrane and almost entirely reabsorbed. A small amount passes through to the urine, but this is considered normal. Results from a reagent strip test are generally reported as negative through 4+ (see Table 5.4). There is another test to detect the presence of total protein in urine which will be discussed later in this chapter.

Table 5.3. Screening Procedures for Orthostatic Proteinuria.

1. Have the patient collect a urine specimen in a clean dry container on rising in the morning.
2. Collect a second specimen in a clean dry container after being up for several hours.
3. Perform a protein determination on both specimens.

Interpretation:
Negative protein in the first specimen and positive protein in the second specimen is indicative of orthostatic proteinuria.

Unit 5

Table 5.4. Protein Reagent* Strip Test Results.

Negative	0 mg/dl
Trace	5–<30 mg/dl
+	30 mg/dl
++	100 mg/dl
+++	300 mg/dl
++++	>2000 mg/dl

*Ames Multistix.

BLOOD

The presence of blood in the urine can take one of two forms, intact red blood cells or free **hemoglobin.** Intact red blood cells is referred to as **hematuria,** and free hemoglobin in the urine is referred to as **hemoglobinuria.** The presence of blood in either form may be significant; this should be noted and the cause investigated.

Hematuria results from bleeding into the renal system at any point from the glomerulus to the urethra. A small number of red blood cells is considered normal. However, any amount detectable on the reagent pad cannot be ignored.

The presence of hemoglobin in the urine can result from the lysing of intact red cells in the urogenital system or from hemoglobin being filtered across the glomerular membrane as a result of intravascular hemolysis. (See Table 5.5 to compare the various sources of red cells and hemoglobin presence in urine.)

The presence of blood in urine can easily be detected with a reagent test strip that contains a hemoglobin detecting pad. The test pad area contains a peroxide and a **chromagen,** which acts as a color indicator. When blood or hemoglobin in urine contacts the pad, it reacts with the peroxide. Oxygen is released and reacts with the chromagen, thus resulting in a color change. If intact red cells are present, they are first lysed on the reagent pad to free the hemoglobin and allow the reaction to proceed. Results are either reported on a scale of negative to large or negative to trace to one plus (+) through three plus (+++).

The laboratory worker needs to be aware of interfering substances. **Myoglobin** is one such substance that contains hemoglobin molecules, but the source is muscle tissue rather than blood. The presence of myoglobin may or may not be significant in itself, but it will cause false-positive reactions with the hemoglobin reagent pad. One way to distinguish myoglobin from hemoglobin is a precipitation test. Hemoglobin will be precipitated after the addition of ammonium sulfate to the urine, whereas myoglobin will not.

Table 5.5. Sources of Blood in the Urine.

Hematuria	Hemoglobinuria
Kidney damage due to trauma	Strenuous exercise
Glomerulonephritis	Transfusion reactions
Pyelonephritis	Hemolytic anemias
Strenuous exercise	Bacterial infections
Bladder infection (cystitis)	Extreme burns
Calculi (kidney stones)	
Tumors	
Kidney damage due to drugs or toxins	

Chemical Examination of Urine

Several causes for false-negative urinary blood results exist. Ascorbic acid (vitamin C) at higher doses than those considered normal will cause false-negative reactions. A specimen which is not well mixed at the time of testing will allow intact red blood cells to settle and not be present in the supernatant. Thus these cells go undetected on the reagent strip. Therefore, specimens must be well mixed prior to testing. False-negative results may be encountered whenever anything prevents the lysis of intact red blood cells. This includes high protein and high specific gravity in combination with low pH.

False-positive results are seen with urine contaminated with menstrual blood; therefore, it is important that urines be properly collected to avoid this type of contamination. Urines from patients with urinary tract infections may also exhibit a false-positive blood reaction. In this case it is important to closely examine urine microscopically for blood if there is a presence of bacteria. A further cause of false-positive results occurs when blood has settled to the bottom of the container. Therefore, it is very important to mix the urine specimen prior to performing the dipstick procedure.

NITRITE

A common problem encountered in the urogenital system is the urinary tract infection (UTI). One screening test for UTI is the nitrite test on the chemical reagent strip used in urinalysis. When gram-negative bacteria are present in the urine, they can convert nitrate, a normal constituent of urine, into nitrite. Nitrite, in turn, reacts with an aromatic amine to form a diazonium salt which changes the color of the reagent pad from white to pink. Results are reported as positive or negative; there is no quantitative or semiquantitative designation as in several other chemical tests. Any positive reaction is considered significant.

Unfortunately, as in most other tests, there are things that may cause false-negative as well as false-positive results. A false-negative result can occur if the specimen is not collected with the correct timing. Urine needs to be held in the bladder at least 4 hours, in order for the bacteria to convert nitrate to nitrite. Therefore, the first morning specimen is the specimen of choice to screen for nitrites. Other causes of false-negative results include bacterial infection by other than gram-negative bacteria. These are still serious infections but will not be detected by the nitrite test. An additional false-negative result is seen when the urine is not tested within 2 hours of collection or is not stored properly. This may allow the nitrite to be further converted to nitrogen by bacteria. Nitrogen will not react with the nitrite-detecting reagents. A false-negative result may also be caused by a diet that does not contain nitrates or is high in ascorbic acid. Nitrates are found in green vegetables. Diets deficient in green vegetables will not provide sufficient nitrate for bacteria to convert into nitrites.

False-positive results are seen when the urine is allowed to stand for too long at room temperature and contaminating bacteria proliferate and convert nitrate into nitrite. This illustrates the importance of proper specimen collection as well as of handling and storage of urine specimens prior to testing. Finally, a false-positive result may occur when the specimen is red in color from some other source. This red color is absorbed by the reagent pad and may appear as a positive reaction. Fortunately, there are other tests that screen for UTI such as the microscopic examination for white blood cells and bacteria (Unit 6), as well as the chemical test for leukocyte esterase.

LEUKOCYTES

Another indicator of UTI is the presence of leukocytes, a type of white blood cell. **Granulated leukocytes** possess granules that contain an **enzyme** compound known as esterase. Esterase can be detected with a chemical reagent strip; in combination with the nitrite test this can provide additional information regarding the presence of UTI. Lymphocytes, which do not contain granules, will not be detected with this test. However, it is granulocytes that are most often present during UTI. Occasionally white blood cells will lyse, thus making it impossible to detect them microscopically; however, with the leukocyte test the technician can still detect their presence.

On the chemical pad, the esterase will react with an ester compound to form an alcohol which in turn reacts with a diazo salt to form a diazo dye. The resultant dye is purple in color and indicates a positive reaction. As with many other tests, this is only a screening test and not quantitative. The results are reported as positive or negative (some manufacturers may grade the positive).

False-positive results can be caused by oxidizing reagents such as chlorine bleach or specimens contaminated with vaginal secretions. False-negative results can be caused by high glucose or high specific gravity. Additionally, certain antibiotics as well as ascorbic acid can cause false-negative results.

KETONES

The detection of ketones in the urine is important in the early diagnosis and monitoring of diabetes mellitus. Ketones are a result of fat metabolism common in diabetics who lack insulin. Insulin allows **carbohydrates** to leave the bloodstream and be utilized. However, if the body cannot have access to carbohydrates, it metabolizes fat as an energy source. Ketones are a product of fat metabolism. These ketones are then used as a source of energy, with the excess being excreted in the urine. A serious consequence of excess ketones, or ketosis, is that it can lead to metabolic acidosis, resulting in coma and even death. Normal urine has a small amount of ketones present. However, this amount is below the sensitivity level of the reagent test strip.

Ketones are also present in other conditions that deprive the patient of carbohydrates, such as starvation. Severe vomiting is another condition in which the body does not get a chance to absorb the carbohydrates that are consumed. Finally, malabsorption, which prevents the body from absorbing carbohydrates, will result in increased fat metabolism.

Ketones are actually a mixture of three different ketones—acetone, acetoacetic acid, and β-hydroxybutyric acid. They are present in the following percentages of total ketones—2%, 20%, and 78%, respectively. The reagent test pad detects primarily the presence of acetoacetic acid. This poses no problem, since the other two ketones are derived from this one. The reagent pad is impregnated with sodium nitroprusside and an alkaline buffer to maintain the proper testing pH. Acetoacetic acid reacts with the sodium nitroprusside to produce a color change. This is sometimes referred to as Legal's test. Results are reported as negative to large, or semiquantitatively as negative to 160 mg/dl.

False positives in ketone analysis are most often associated with antibiotics and other medications that will react with the reagent pad. False-positive results can also be seen with highly pigmented urines that may mask the reagent pad

Chemical Examination of Urine

and with improperly stored specimens in which the ketones have been allowed to evaporate out of the urine.

GLUCOSE

One of the most important chemical urine tests is the one for glucose. Glucose present in the urine, termed **glycosuria** or **glucosuria,** may be an indication of diabetes mellitus. It should be pointed out that glycosuria is not diagnostic for diabetes mellitus but rather is an important indicator. Urine analysis in conjunction with other tests such as the blood glucose level, the glucose tolerance test, and the presence of ketones in the blood and urine are used to diagnose diabetes mellitus.

The blood glucose level in normal individuals is approximately 70 to 110 mg/dl. This may be as high as 160 mg/dl following a meal high in carbohydrates. All blood glucose is filtered across the glomerular membrane but is reabsorbed in the proximal convoluted tubule. However, the proximal convoluted tubule cannot reabsorb glucose with a concentration greater than approximately 180 mg/dl. The excess "spills over" into the urine and can be detected with the glucose pad on the reagent test strip. Another cause of glucose in the urine includes a defect in the reabsorbing tubule; thus glycosuria can be present with a normal blood glucose level. By far the predominant cause of glycosuria is diabetes mellitus.

The chemical reagent strip test used to detect glucose in urine is based on the reagent glucose oxidase. This, plus peroxidase and a chromagen, a color indicator, results in a color change in the pad that is directly proportional to the amount of glucose in the urine.

Results can be reported on a plus scale (negative to 4+), or semiquantitatively from negative to 2000 mg/dl. The reagent pad will not detect the presence of other sugars, such as galactose, which may be diagnostic of disease. However, there is a confirmatory test which can detect other sugars and will be discussed later in this unit.

As with other reagent strip tests, ascorbic acid can cause false-negative reactions. False-negative readings can also be caused by improperly stored specimens or those with a high bacterial presence. The bacteria will consume the glucose for their own metabolism. Therefore, improperly stored specimens in which bacteria have proliferated may yield a false-negative result. False-positive readings are less common and usually associated with an improperly collected specimen.

BILIRUBIN AND UROBILINOGEN

Bilirubin and urobilinogen are two breakdown products of hemoglobin. When red cells are removed from circulation, the hemoglobin is released back into the circulation, where it is converted to bilirubin. This bilirubin is water insoluble, bound to albumin, and referred to unconjugated bilirubin. In this form it cannot cross the glomerular membrane. In the liver, the bilirubin is released from albumin and bound to glucuronic acid, making it water soluble. It is now referred to as conjugated bilirubin. At this point the conjugated bilirubin is secreted via the bile duct into the small intestine, where it is converted into urobilinogen. If unconjugated bilirubin is allowed to build up in the plasma, this may lead to a condition known as **jaundice.** The majority of urobilinogen is expelled in the feces, but approximately 20% is reabsorbed into the bloodstream. Most of the reabsorbed compound returns to the liver where it is reexcreted, but a small por-

```
Hemoglobin        ⎤
    ↓             ⎬ Blood and reticuloendothelial system
Unconjugated      ⎦
bilirubin         ⎤
    ↓             ⎬ Liver
Conjugated        ⎦
bilirubin
    ↓
Urobilinogen      ⎤
    ↓             ⎬ Intestine
Feces             ⎦
```

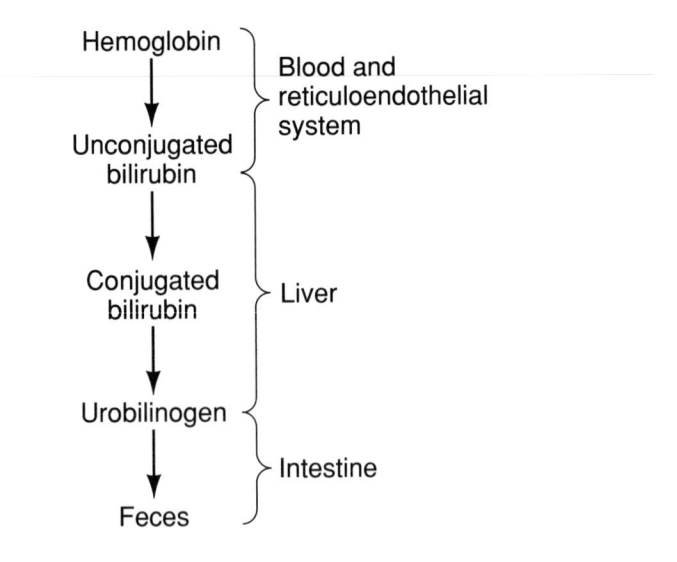

fig. 5.1. Normal Metabolism of Hemoglobin.

tion crosses the glomerular membrane and is excreted in the urine. (See Figure 5.1 for a diagram of normal bilirubin and urobilinogen metabolism.)

In normal urine, the amount of bilirubin and urobilinogen is not detectable by routine testing methods. However, certain conditions will cause an increase in bilirubin, urobilinogen, or both in the urine. (See Table 5.6 for a summary of the causes of altered bilirubin metabolism.)

Urinary Bilirubin Detection

A significant increase in the amount of bilirubin in urine will result in a urine with a distinct amber or dark-yellow color. If the urine is shaken vigorously, a yellow foam will appear. Although bilirubin may not be present in sufficient amounts to create the above results, it could still be significant. There is a chemical test for bilirubin that can be performed using a reagent strip. Bilirubin will react with a diazonium salt to form a dye which will result in a color change in the reagent pad ranging from light brown or tan to a darker tan or pink color. Results may be reported from negative to large or from negative to 3+.

False-positive results may be seen in any condition in which the urine has pigment that will change the color of the pad. Ascorbic acid can be a cause of false-

Table 5.6. Causes of Variant Bilirubin/Urobilinogen Results and Resulting Urine Findings.

	Bilirubin	**Urobilinogen**
Prehepatic		
Transfusion reactions		
Inherited and acquired anemias	Negative	Increased
Sickle cell disease		
Hepatic		
Cirrhosis		
Hepatitis	Increased	Normal to increased
Liver trauma		
Posthepatic		
Calculi obstruction of bile duct	Increased	Normal*
Tumor obstruction of bile duct		

*It appears normal on the dipstick, but it is actually absent.

Chemical Examination of Urine

negative readings. Another cause of a false-negative result could be the prolonged exposure of urine containing bilirubin to light. This degrades the bilirubin, rendering it nonreactive with the reagent pad. Once again, the importance of proper collection and storage is illustrated.

Urinary Urobilinogen Testing

As discussed earlier, urobilinogen is normally present in a small amount in urine. Therefore, detection tests must be able to detect significant amounts while "ignoring" the normal amount. There are two primary methods for detecting urobilinogen in urine, depending on which manufacturer's reagent strip test is used. The Ames Multistix reaction is based on urobilinogen reacting with Ehrlich's reagent, which generates a color reaction that can be noted on the reagent pad. Ehrlich's reagent is actually *p*-dimethylaminobenzaldehyde and named after the originator of the test. Unfortunately there are many compounds that will react with Ehrlich's reagent that will result in a false-positive reaction. Chemstrip utilizes a diazonium salt that is specific for urobilinogen and results in dye production that changes the color of the reagent pad. Results are reported as normal (0.2 to 1.0 mg/dl) to several mg/dl of urobilinogen. Results may be reported as Ehrlich units as follows: 1 Ehrlich unit is equal to 1.0 mg/dl of urine. Since this reagent is more specific for urobilinogen, fewer false-positive reactions are found. However, any-

---

EXERCISE 25 — FALSE-POSITIVE AND FALSE-NEGATIVE REACTIONS

The instructor should organize the class into small groups. The groups should be instructed to:

Construct a table listing the causes of false-positive and false-negative results for each chemical test.

EXERCISE 26 — CHEMICAL TESTS

The instructor should have each student:

1. Select a chemical test.
2. Do further reading on the test.
3. Prepare a 5- to 10-minute discussion of the test.
4. Present their report before the class.

The instructor should:

5. Conduct a question and answer session for the reports.

EXERCISE 27: URINARY CHEMICAL TESTING

The students should wear gloves, goggles, and face shields for this exercise. The instructor should provide each student with a urine specimen and a worksheet. The students should be instructed to:

1. Select a chemical reagent strip.
2. Record the lot number and expiration date.
3. Perform the dipstick procedure on the urine provided.
4. Record the results on their worksheet.
5. Trade their urine specimen with a fellow student and repeat the procedure.
6. Complete 5 urinalyses.
7. Turn in their worksheet.

The instructor should check their work.

---

thing that may cause a color change in the reagent pad could mask the presence of urobilinogen. False-negative results may occur with improper storage of the specimen and the presence of ascorbic acid or high levels of nitrite.

SPECIFIC GRAVITY

Whereas specific gravity is traditionally considered a physical property of urine, it is possible to measure the specific gravity with a chemical reagent strip. (See Unit 4 for a review.)

CONFIRMATORY AND SUPPLEMENTARY TESTS

Whereas the above section discussed the various tests that may be done with a reagent strip, occasionally the results obtained must be confirmed or verified. This section will discuss the most common confirmatory tests.

PROTEIN PRECIPITATION TEST

Occasionally the reagent strip test for protein will be inconclusive and a confirmatory test must be performed. The most common one for protein is the sulfosalicylic acid (SSA) precipitation test. Since the chemical reagent strip test is primarily sensitive to albumin, other forms of protein may go undetected. The SSA test will precipitate all forms of protein. A good example of this is when the reagent strip is negative and the SSA is positive due to the presence of Bence-Jones protein. This is a low molecular weight protein associated with some forms of multiple myeloma. However, a definitive diagnosis of multiple myeloma and Bence-Jones protein would be by electrophoresis.

Chemical Examination of Urine

The principal reagent, usually 3% or 7% weight/volume (w/v) sulfosalicylic acid, will precipitate all protein in urine. It is very important to use the supernatant of centrifuged urine, because this is clear. It should be mixed in equal volume with the sulfosalicylic acid. The precipitation is graded from negative (no precipitation) to 4+ (see Table 5.7). Additionally, some laboratories will set up standards with known concentrations of protein for comparison to the SSA test. This allows the technician to more accurately quantify the amount of protein in the urine.

False-negative reactions may occur when a highly alkaline urine is tested. The alkalinity may neutralize the acid, rendering it unable to precipitate protein. False-positive results may occur if there is a high concentration of antibiotics such as penicillin or radiographic dyes.

COPPER REDUCTION TESTS FOR SUGAR

Occasionally the need arises for urine to be tested for the presence of sugars other than glucose. For example, newborns with an inborn error of metabolism that prevents them from metabolizing galactose will develop **galactosemia** and **galactosuria.** This would not be detected using a reagent chemistry strip which is only sensitive to glucose. The copper reduction test will, however, detect galactose in the urine. Each laboratory will establish their own protocol; however, generally all children under 2 to 3 years of age should have this test done whenever a urinalysis is performed.

Clinitest (Miles, Inc.) is the tablet form of the copper reduction test. This test requires that 5 drops of urine be mixed with 10 drops of water and that one Clinitest tablet be added. The reaction is based on a reducing substance, the sugar, reacting with cupric sulfate to form cuprous oxide. This results in color change from blue (negative) to green, yellow, and orange (strong positive), depending on the amount of reducing substance present.

This test is not as sensitive as the reagent dipstick for glucose. Therefore, it is not a true confirmatory test. A technician can obtain a positive reagent strip test and a negative Clinitest. However, it is also possible to have a positive Clinitest and a negative dipstick. This indicates that possibly some other reducing sugar is present. This is when the Clinitest is most helpful. It should be noted that table sugar or sucrose is not a reducing sugar.

False-positive reactions are seen when a nonsugar reducing substance, such as ascorbic acid or certain antibiotics, is present. False-negative results are seen when "pass through" occurs. This happens when a very large amount of reducing substance is present and the reaction "passes through" the color range very quickly and returns to what appears to be the original negative color. This is why it is very important to follow directions carefully and read the test at the proper time interval. One note of caution: Do not hold the test tube while the reaction

Table 5.7. Protein Sulfosalicylic Acid Precipitation Test.

Negative	No visible precipitation	0 mg/dl
Trace	Slight turbidity	5–<30 mg/dl
+	Distinct turbidity; cannot read print through solution	30 mg/dl
++	Turbidity with granulation	100 mg/dl
+++	Turbidity with granulation and flocculation	300 mg/dl
++++	Large or solid clumps of precipitation	>500 mg/dl

• Unit 5

is occurring! The reaction generates heat, which could burn you. Place the test tube in a rack and observe the reaction. You may pick the test tube up by the rim to compare it to the reaction chart.

BILIRUBIN CONFIRMATION TEST

The Ictotest (Miles, Inc., Elkhart, IN) is truly a confirmatory test for the presence of bilirubin. It is more sensitive than the reagent chemistry strip. Therefore, when a technician gets a positive result using the dipstick, the Ictotest is used to confirm the presence or absence of bilirubin.

The test involves the same reagents as the dipstick but utilizes a larger pad. (See Table 5.8 for the Ictotest procedure.)

INSTRUMENTATION

Whenever a urinalysis is performed by a technician, there is the possibility of error due to individual variation. Slight differences occur between technicians with regard to the timing of reading the specimen. There is also variation regarding color interpretation. The introduction of instrumentation into the urinalysis procedure can control variation in the timing and color interpretation of the chemistry reagent strip (see Figure 5.2).

Table 5.8. Ictotest Procedure.

1. Ten drops of urine are placed on the Ictotest pad (any bilirubin present is concentrated on the surface of the pad while the remaining urine is absorbed into the pad).
2. An Ictotest tablet is then placed on the pad and drops of water are added.
3. The tablet is removed after 30 seconds and the pad is observed for color.
4. A purple or blue test indicates a positive reaction; any other color is considered negative. (The same interferences that may confound the dipstick test also may interfere with this test.)

EXERCISE 28 INVESTIGATING CONFIRMATORY TESTS

It is recommended that 1 week be given for this assignment. In small groups, the students should:

1. Contact local hospitals to find out which confirmatory or supplementary tests they perform. (This may be the hospital where they will be doing their clinical practicum.)
2. Discover under what circumstances the laboratories perform the tests.
3. Prepare a report.
4. Present the report before the class.

Chemical Examination of Urine

EXERCISE 29 CONFIRMATORY TESTING

The students should wear gloves, goggles, and face shields for this exercise. The instructor should provide each student with a urine specimen and a worksheet. The instructor should tell the students to:

1. Perform a reagent strip urinalysis.
2. Determine if any confirmatory testing needs to be done.
3. Complete any necessary confirmatory testing.
4. Trade with a fellow student and repeat the exercise.

The instructor should check the results.

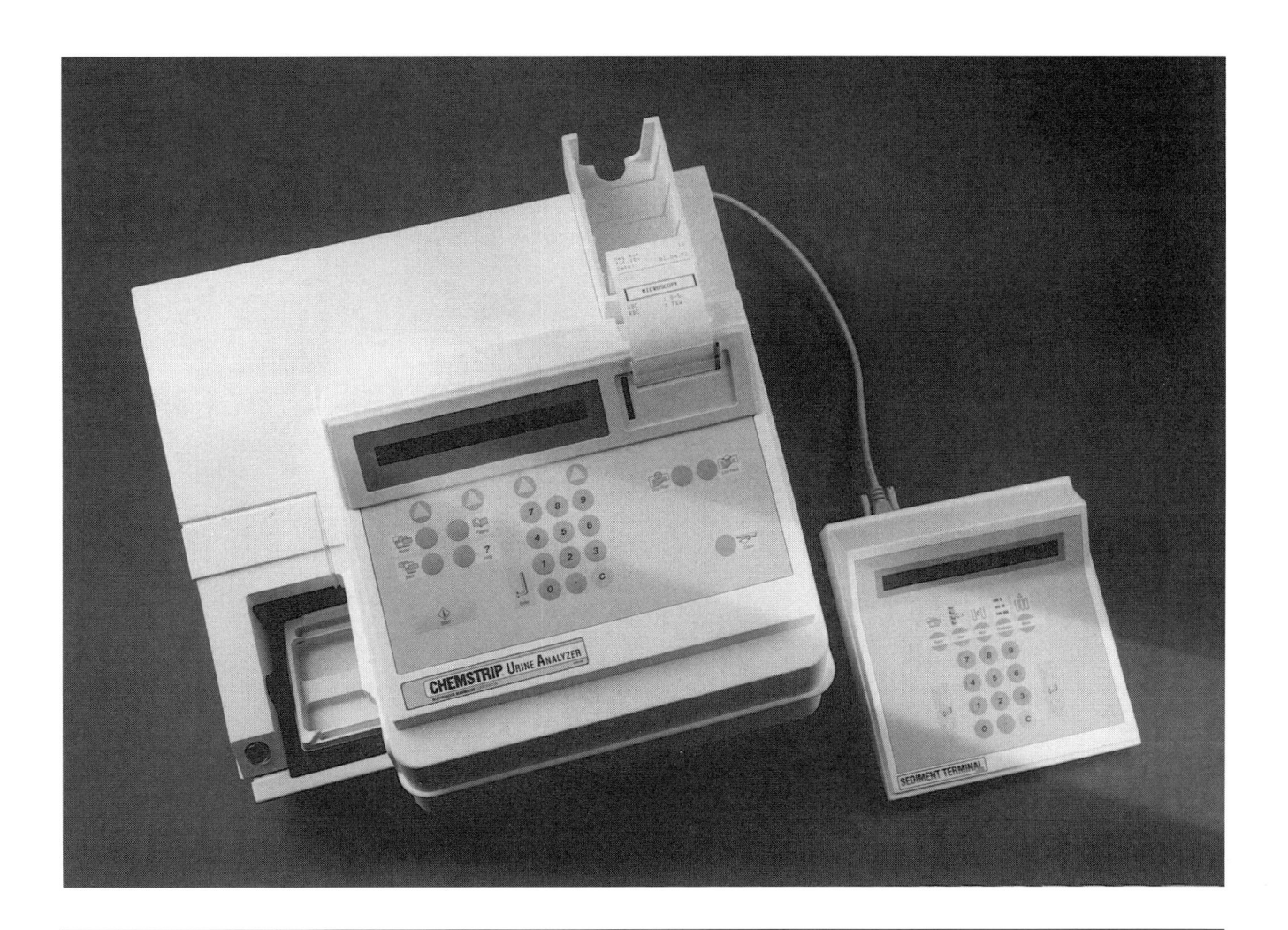

fig. 5.2. The Chemstrip Automated Urine Analyzer (Boehringer Mannheim Corp., Indianapolis, IN).

Unit 5

There are several instruments available for use in urinalysis (see Table 5.9). However, all instruments operate on the principle of light reflection. The reagent strips are dipped in the urine as previously described and placed on the instrument reader. As the concentration of an analyte increases or causes the reagent pad to change color, the amount of reflected light from the pad changes. The pads are consistently read at the appropriate time. The amount of light reflected from each pad is compared with known internal instrument concentrations; therefore, the urine chemical concentrations can be calculated and displayed. This eliminates the possibility of technician variation.

Table 5.9. Urinalysis Instrumentation.

Instrument	Manufacturer
Chemstrip Urine Analyzer	Boehringer Mannheim Corp.
Clinitek 100 Urine Chemistry Analyzer	Miles, Inc.
Clinitek 200+ Urine Chemistry Analyzer	Miles, Inc.
Rapimat II	Behring Diagnostics

EXERCISE 30 URINALYSIS INSTRUMENTATION

In small groups, the instructor should have the students:

1. Research a piece of instrumentation used for urinalysis. This should include cost, ease of use, technology, and quality control requirements.
2. Prepare an overhead which summarizes their findings.
3. Present this in class.

SUMMARY

As initially discussed, the reagent strip test for the chemical analysis of urine is a very simple test to perform. However, as can be seen in this chapter, there is a wealth of information that can be obtained as long as manufacturer's directions are closely followed and the technician is aware of possible interfering substances. The next chapter will discuss the microscopic analysis of urine which often accompanies and complements the chemical analysis of urine.

REVIEW QUESTIONS

1. This test is based on the reaction of hydrogen ions with color indicators.
   a. blood
   b. pH ✓
   c. specific gravity
   d. white blood cells

2. Which of the following is the best way to perform the dipstick procedure?
   a. dipping the dipstick, then standing it upright so that the color change can be observed
   b. submerging the dipstick in the urine for 1 minute, then removing and comparing with color chart
   c. quickly submerging then removing dipstick from the urine in a way to remove excess urine, then placing horizontally ✓
   d. all of the above are acceptable

3. Multiple myeloma is a condition that results in the increased production of
   a. blood
   b. ketones
   c. nitrite
   d. protein ✓

4. This substance will give false-positive reactions with the hemoglobin detection reagent pad.
   a. albumin
   b. bacteria
   c. myoglobin ✓
   d. red blood cells

5. The detection of this substance is based upon a test known as the _____ error of indicators.
   a. blood
   b. ketones
   c. nitrite
   d. protein ✓

Match the primary reagent with the proper urine constituent.
6. Nitrite   b   a. hydrogen peroxide
7. Bilirubin e   b. aromatic amine
8. Ketone   d   c. glucose oxidase
9. Glucose   c   d. sodium nitroprusside
10. Blood   a   e. diazonium salt

Unit 5

11. An Ehrlich unit is a unit of measurement for which chemical constituent?
    a. bilirubin
    b. ketones
    c. nitrite
    d. urobilinogen

12. Galactose can be detected with which test?
    a. Clinitest
    b. Ictotest
    c. Salicylate precipitation test
    d. none of the above

13. Blockage of the bile duct will result in an increase of this in urine.
    a. bilirubin
    b. hemoglobin
    c. nitrite
    d. urobilinogen

14. This is a screen for urinary tract infections.
    a. bilirubin
    b. ketones
    c. leukocyte esterase
    d. pH

15. Which of the following are good screening tests for diabetes mellitus?
    a. bilirubin/urobilinogen
    b. ketones/glucose
    c. nitrite/leukocyte esterase
    d. blood/specific gravity

UNIT 6

Microscopic Examination of Urine

LEARNING OBJECTIVES

After studying this unit, it is the responsibility of the student to know the following objectives:

- Define all terms listed in the glossary.

- Name and state the function of all parts of the microscope.

- Calculate the total magnification for given lens specifications.

- Follow the proper procedure for microscopic examination of prepared slides and wet preparations of urine sediment.

- Demonstrate proper care and storage of the microscope.

- Outline the general procedure for performing a microscopic examination of urine.

- List and identify by sight formed elements in a urinary sediment.

- Describe the clinical significance of each formed element found in urinary sediment.

GLOSSARY

amorphous phosphates crystalline precipitate of a phosphate salt having no distinguishable shape or form.

amorphous urates crystalline precipitate of a uric acid salt having no distinguishable shape or form.

binocular having two oculars or eyepieces.

condenser microscope part which directs the light onto the viewed object.

hematuria presence of blood or hemoglobin in the urine.

iatrogenic as a result of treatment.

interpupillary distance distance between the eyepiece tubes.

iris diaphragm adjustment in the condenser of a microscope to regulate the amount of light striking the viewed object.

monocular having one ocular or eyepiece.

objectives magnifying lens on the microscope.

ocular microscope eyepiece which contains a magnifying lens.

oval fat bodies renal tubule epithelial cell or macrophage with ingested fat.

parfocal ability to change from one objective to another without losing focus of the object.

pyuria presence of white cells in the urine.

renal epithelial cells cells originating in the renal tubules.

revolving nosepiece turning plate on which the objectives are attached.

squamous epithelial cells cells which line the lower portions of the genitourinary tract.

supravital stain used to stain living cells.

Tamm-Horsfall protein high molecular weight mucoprotein secreted by the renal tubules.

total magnification product of the magnifying power of the ocular and the objective of a microscope.

transitional epithelial cells cells between the pelvis of the kidney and the base of the bladder.

urinary sediment formed elements of a urine which have been condensed during centrifugation.

working distance distance between the bottom of the objective and the object being viewed when in sharp focus.

INTRODUCTION

The practice of urinalysis involves the physical and chemical analysis discussed in previous units. Additionally, a microscopic examination of urine is performed to enable the technician to visualize and quantitate the formed elements or solid material contained in the urine.

This unit will include basic information on use of the microscope and specific details on the formed elements found in the urine. In addition, the quantitation and identification of the formed elements will be discussed.

USE OF THE MICROSCOPE

The microscope is a valuable piece of equipment in the urinalysis laboratory. It is used to visualize cellular items too small to be seen by the naked eye. Each technician must have an understanding of the parts and workings of the light microscope. Experience in light microscopy will be imperative. Additionally, the proper care and storage of the microscope is required to achieve consistently accurate results when performing microscopic urinalysis.

PARTS OF THE MICROSCOPE

The parts and their function will be similar for each microscope, regardless of the style or manufacturer of the instrument. Arrangement and placement of the parts will vary. In order to aid in understanding, the major parts will be discussed in related groups.

Magnification

The **oculars,** or eyepieces, are located at the top of the microscope (see Figure 6.1). Each ocular contains a lens that magnifies the image on the slide. When two oculars are present, as in Figure 6.1, the microscope is **binocular,** whereas a microscope with one ocular is **monocular.** The majority of laboratory microscopes are binocular. When a binocular microscope is used, the oculars must be adjusted to the proper **interpupillary distance** for each user. This is usually done by adjusting a thumbscrew near the oculars.

Additional magnification is found in the **objectives** (see Figure 6.1). The objectives are attached to the **revolving nosepiece.** Like the oculars, each objective has a lens for magnification. The number of objectives on a microscope is usually three. Each objective is marked on the exterior with a color and the degree of magnification. The low-power objective is most often 10X. This indicates that it magnifies ten times the size of the object. The high-power, or high-dry, objective will frequently be 40X. The most powerful magnifying objective is the oil-immersion objective, which is most often 100X. For microscopic urinalysis, the low- and high-power objectives are used.

To obtain an understanding of the magnifying power of any microscope, the concept of **total magnification** is important. As described above, two magnifying lenses, the ocular and objective, are in use when viewing an object. It is the product of these two lenses that provides the total magnifying power for the

■ Unit 6

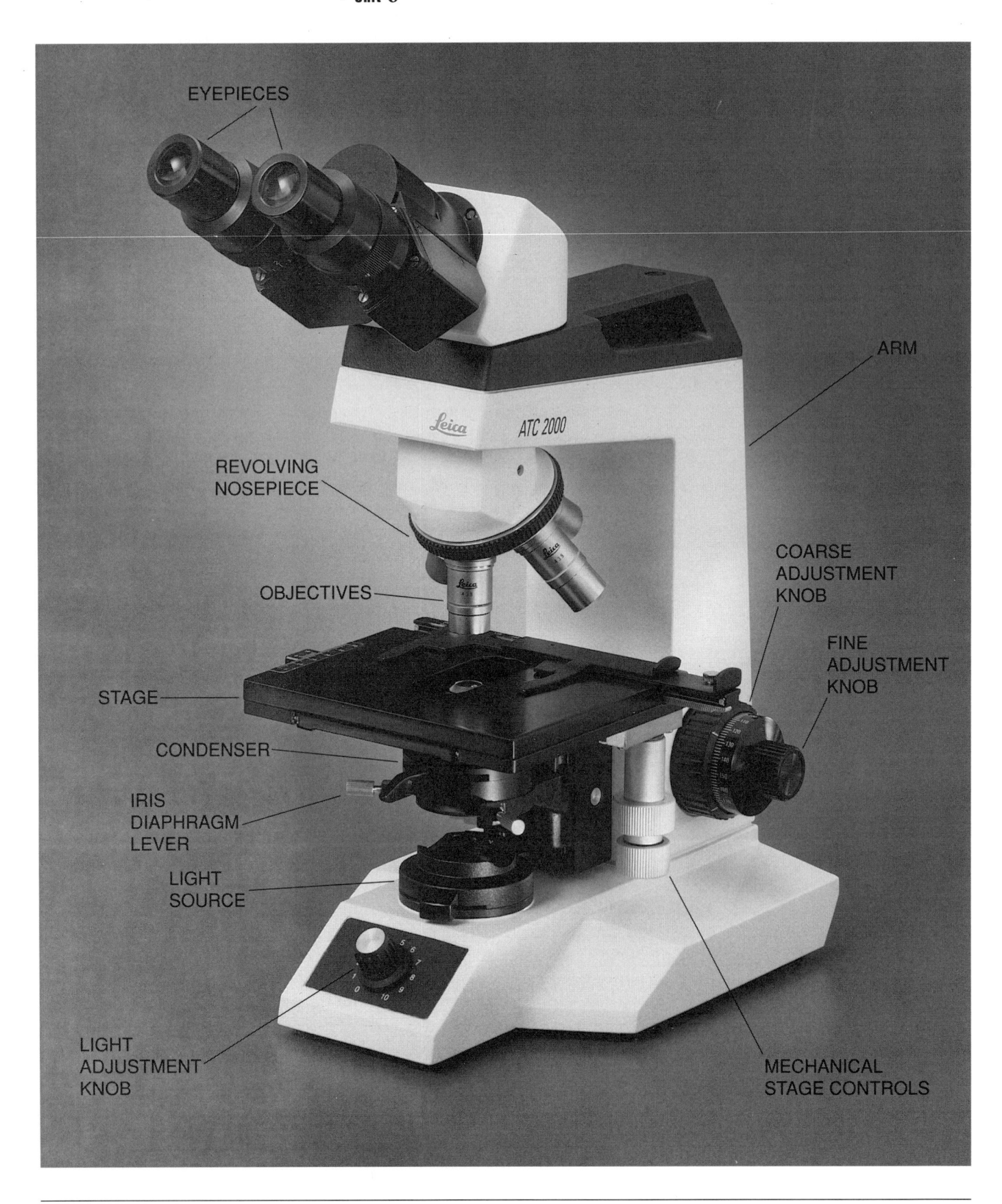

fig. 6.1. Binocular microscope. (Courtesy of Leica, Inc., Buffalo, N.Y.)

Microscopic Examination of Urine

microscope. For example, if the microscope has a 10X ocular and a 40x high-power objective in use, the total magnification will be:

$$(10x) \times (40x) = 400x$$

Therefore, any object viewed with this combination of lenses will be magnified 400 times its size.

Coarse and Fine Focus Adjustments

Coarse and fine focus adjustments are located near the base of the microscope (see Figure 6.1). These adjustments permit the focusing of the object being viewed. Both knobs cause movement of either the nosepiece or the stage, depending on the microscope.

The coarse adjustment is the largest knob. It permits movement over large distances and should be used only when the low-power objective is in place. This is to prevent damage to the objective as well as to the object being viewed. The coarse adjustment is used for the initial focusing.

Once the object is brought into view using the coarse adjustment, the fine focus adjustment may be used to provide a sharper focus. This feature creates movement over small distances and may be used with any objective.

Initial focusing of any object may be done only in low power. The change to high-power and then oil-immersion objectives may follow. It is important that the object remain in focus when switching from one objective to another. When this can be done, the microscope is said to be **parfocal.**

What prevents the use of the coarse focus with the high-power or oil-immersion objective is the **working distance** with each of these objectives. The working distance is the distance between the bottom of the objective and the top of the object being viewed. When the high-dry and oil-immersion objectives are in place, this distance is very small. There is little margin for movement of the objective. The low-power objective has a much greater working distance and therefore can be used with the coarse adjustment.

Illumination

Illumination of the viewed object is provided by parts located on the base and under the stage of the microscope (see Figure 6.1). The major illumination is the light source. It is located on the base of the microscope and contains a lamp that provides the source of the light. The intensity of the light may be regulated by an

EXERCISE 31 DETERMINATION OF MAGNIFICATION

Each student should obtain a microscope and perform the following:

1. Identify the oculars and objectives.
2. Determine the magnification of the oculars and each objective.
3. Calculate the total magnification when each objective is used with the oculars.
4. Adjust the interpupillary distance and note the setting for future use.

▪ Unit 6

adjustment knob located on or near the source. The remainder of the parts are involved with directing and regulating the amount of light from the source.

The **condenser** is located above the light source and serves to direct light to the objective. The condenser may be raised or lowered by using the condenser adjustment knob located on the arm of the microscope (see Figure 6.1). Raising the condenser will increase the illumination directed to the objective and the object will appear brighter. Lowering the condenser will have the reverse effect.

The **iris diaphragm** is located in the condenser. It regulates the amount of light that strikes the object in view. The amount of light may be regulated by a movable lever (see Figure 6.1).

Light regulation involves proper adjustment of lamp intensity, condenser, and iris diaphragm while focusing the viewed object. The amount of light will vary, depending on the object being viewed.

USE OF THE MICROSCOPE

When using the microscope, the technician should take care to use proper technique. This helps to assure proper results and viewing as well as the comfort of the user.

For the comfort of the technician, the seat should be adjusted to the correct height. The technician should be able to look into the microscope without bending the head down or raising the head to see into the eyepieces. The microscope should be placed directly in front of the viewer with the base close to the edge of the table, but safely secure from falling. The table where the microscope is placed must have an area where individuals can place their legs when sitting. This reduces back and neck strain.

When carrying the microscope, always use two hands. One hand should carry the microscope by the arm (see Figure 6.2), while the second hand is placed under the base for support.

EXERCISE 32 IDENTIFICATION OF MICROSCOPE PARTS

Each student should obtain a microscope and identify the following parts:

1. Coarse and fine focus knobs.
2. Condenser.
3. Light source.
4. Iris diaphragm.

These identified parts should be checked by the instructor.

Microscopic Examination of Urine ▪

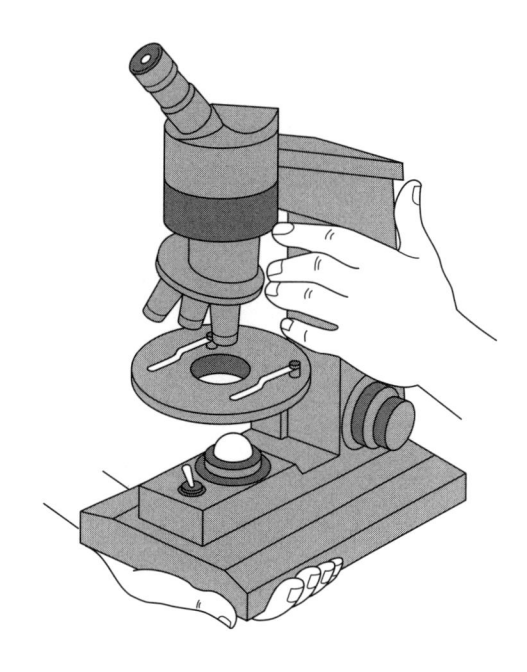

fig. 6.2. The proper method of transporting a microscope.

EXERCISE 33 USE OF THE MICROSCOPE

For this exercise each student should have the following equipment:

1. A compound microscope with cover.
2. Prepared slides.
3. Lens paper.
4. Immersion oil.

Using the equipment above, each student should complete the following exercise. The student should be certain to refer to Figure 6.1 for identification of microscope parts.

Procedure:

1. Obtain a prepared stained slide of either blood cells or bacteria from the instructor.
2. Clean the oculars with lens paper.
3. Adjust the interpupillary distance to the setting determined previously.
4. Place the slide on the stage and secure with the stage clips.
5. Turn on the light source and place at a setting midway on the dial.
6. Move the condenser halfway up.

EXERCISE 33: USE OF THE MICROSCOPE *continued*

7. Open the iris diaphragm about halfway.

Note: At any time the condenser and iris diaphragm may be adjusted to provide more or less light as needed.

8. Rotate the low-power objective into place. Be sure to hear it click.
9. Watching from the side, use the coarse adjustment to move the low-power objective to its lowest position.

Note: Always watch from the side to determine when the objective has stopped moving down.

10. While looking through the oculars, use the coarse adjustment to bring the object into focus.
11. Scan the slide using the low-power objective.
12. On a piece of paper diagram a field.
13. Rotate the high-power objective into place.
14. Looking through the oculars, use the fine adjustment to make the image clearer.

Note: Do *not* use the coarse adjustment. This could damage the objective and/or slide.

15. Diagram a field on a piece of paper.

Note: The oil-immersion objective is not utilized in the urinalysis laboratory and hence will not be used in this exercise.

16. Rotate the low-power objective back into place.
17. Turn off the light source.
18. Remove the slide from the stage.
19. Use lens paper to clean all objectives and oculars.
20. Store the microscope as indicated below.
21. Clean work area and wash hands.

CARE AND STORAGE OF THE MICROSCOPE

An important aspect to successful microscopy is the proper care and storage of the microscope. All working parts must be kept clean and dust free. Immersion oil must be removed entirely from all microscope parts immediately after use.

Upon completion of microscopy, all oculars and objectives must be cleaned with lens paper. The stage should be cleaned with paper tissues. The dustcover must be intact and in place at all times when the microscope is not in use.

Before storage, proper preparation is imperative. The exercise below will outline a protocol for preparation of the microscope for storage.

MICROSCOPIC EXAMINATION OF URINE

Following the preliminary examination steps, which include physical and chemical evaluations, the microscopic examination of the urinary sediment is performed. This microscopic examination is routinely performed on all urines in some laboratories. Other laboratories, however, perform the microscopic examination only when physical and chemical screening tests exhibit positive results.

SPECIMEN COLLECTION AND PREPARATION

In order to obtain an accurate assessment of the urinary sediment, an acceptable specimen must be obtained. The best results arise from a first morning, midstream, clean catch specimen that is examined within 2 hours of collection. Urines that cannot be examined immediately should be refrigerated to preserve the integrity of the microscopic elements.

The microscopic examination is performed on the **urinary sediment**. The urine must be concentrated prior to microscopic examination. It is this concentration step that creates the sediment.

Sedimentation of the urine is done by centrifuging an aliquot of well-mixed urine. In order to obtain a sufficient volume of sediment, 10 to 15 ml of urine is used. This urine is placed in a conical centrifuge tube and centrifuged at 2000 rpm for 5 minutes. Once the urine is centrifuged, the clear supernatant is drained from the concentrated solid material in the bottom of the tube. The supernatant may be decanted into a separate tube for use in chemical confirmatory tests.

EXERCISE 34 STORAGE OF THE MICROSCOPE

After using the microscope, the student should prepare the microscope for storage. Using any microscope, the student should complete the following steps and have the work checked by the instructor.

1. Put low-power objective in place.
2. Move stage clips into a central stage position.
3. Move stage as far back as possible.
4. Clean objectives with lens paper.
5. Clean stage with paper tissues.
6. Unplug and wrap cord around the bottom of arm.
7. Lower condenser to lowest position.
8. Put cover in place.
9. Properly transport microscope to storage area.

Once the supernatant has been decanted, the sediment is mixed by gently resuspending the solid material in the small amount of remaining supernatant urine. A drop of the sediment is used for examination. This drop is placed on a slide or into a counting chamber as designated by the system being used by the laboratory. The drop of urine is examined and the formed elements quantitated.

STANDARDIZATION

Several systems are available for use when examining urinary sediments. These systems are useful because they provide a standardization system. This standardization adds an element of quality assurance each time a urine sediment is examined. The system includes equipment that aids in decanting and standardization of the volume of sediment evaluated on each urine.

Each system provides capped centrifuge tubes, pipettes, standardized slides, and in some cases a **supravital stain.** Systems available include the Kova system (ICL Scientific, Fountain Valley, CA), the UriSystem (Fisher Scientific, Pittsburgh, PA), and Count 6 or Count 10 system (V-Tech, Inc., Palm Desert, CA). For information on any of these systems, the student is referred to the individual company.

MICROSCOPIC TECHNIQUES

Brightfield or light microscopy is the most common method used for examination of the unstained urinary sediment. Although used most often, light microscopy is the most difficult method for viewing the formed elements in the sediment. The light must be reduced to give sufficient contrast to many of the unstained elements. This can be achieved by moving the condenser down about 2 mm and using the iris diaphragm to increase the contrast. It is vital that the contrast be sufficient; if not, some translucent elements such as casts and mucus threads may be missed.

Consistent use of the fine focus adjustment will aid in visualizing items that do not provide a great deal of contrast in the unstained urine. Along with reduced lighting, bringing the field in and out of focus with the fine adjustment will reduce the likelihood that microscopic elements will be missed.

Phase contrast microscopy is very useful for examining urinary sediment. It provides a greater contrast between the formed elements and the background. However, some formed elements are not visible with phase contrast microscopy. Therefore, the ideal situation is a microscope that allows the microscopist to readily change from light to phase.

Polarizing microscopy, although not often readily available, is useful for differentiating elements that polarize light from those that do not. For example, polarizing microscopy is useful for differentiating bacteria from some crystals. If available, polarizing microscopy can be useful in viewing urine sediments.

Urine sediments are usually viewed unstained; however, staining with any of a variety of stains aids in element identification with light microscopy. Supravital stains are available and may be used if desired.

CONSTITUENTS OF A NORMAL URINE SEDIMENT

A normal urine should have very little sediment. There are, however, a few elements that may be found in any urine. These include squamous epithelial cells,

EXERCISE 35 COMPARISON OF TYPES OF MICROSCOPY

Using references provided by the instructor:

1. Research phase and polarizing microscopy.
2. Compare the use of phase and polarizing microscopy to light microscopy in microscopic urinalysis.
3. Create a chart that distinguishes the appearance of microscopic elements in the urine with each type of microscopy.
4. Share the chart with a partner.

especially in women; a very small amount of white or red blood cells; a few hyaline casts; and in some instances crystals that are dependent on dietary constituents. Each laboratory must establish its own normal ranges in accordance with methodology and patient population.

FORMED ELEMENTS IN URINARY SEDIMENT

Cells Found in Sediment

Red Blood Cells. When found in urinary sediment, red blood cells appear much as they do when viewed in peripheral blood. They have the appearance of a biconcave disk that is pale and light refractive (see Figure 6.3). Red cells must be viewed under high power for proper identification. If the urine is not isotonic or does not have the same concentration of particles as the internal contents of the red cells (isotonic), the cells will undergo morphologic changes. The cells may appear swollen or crenated (shrunken). Crenated cells will appear to have spicules around the membrane of the cell. If the cells have been hemolyzed due to the tonicity of the urine, the empty membrane will appear as a ghost cell. Presence of increased numbers of red cells in the urine is termed **hematuria** and often represents a renal disease or damage.

Red blood cells are quantitated in the urine by obtaining an average of cells per high power field (hpf). This is done by observing a minimum of ten fields and averaging the findings.

White Blood Cells. White blood cells may be present in small numbers in a normal urine. As many as five per high power field would not be considered abnormal. These cells enter the urine from secretions of the genital tract or anywhere along the urogenital tract. More than five per high power field may indicate an infection or inflammation at some location along the urinary tract. Infection is particularly suspect if the white blood cells appear along with increased numbers of bacteria. Increased numbers of white blood cells in the urine is termed **pyuria.**

White blood cells appear larger than red blood cells when viewed under high power. They will most often have a visible nucleus and may also have visible

▪ Unit 6

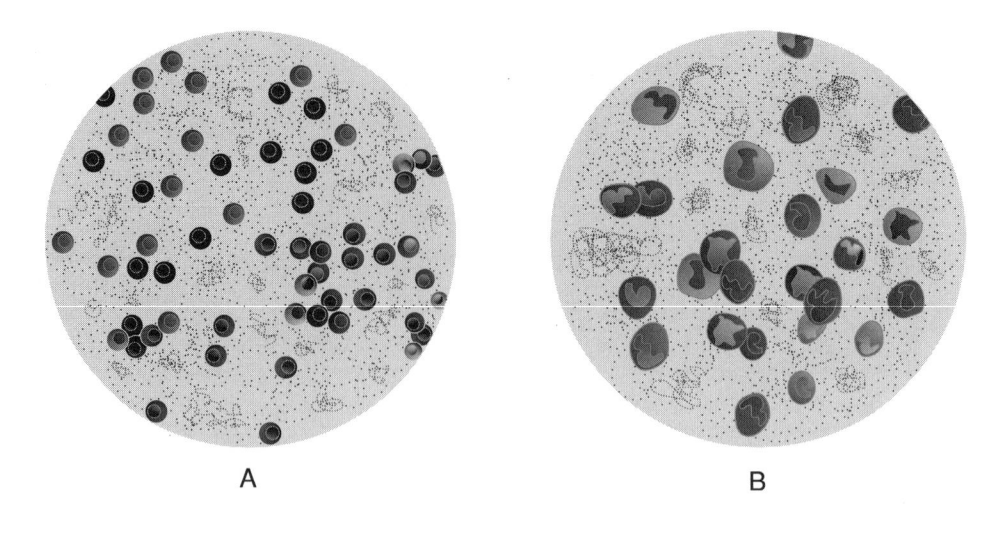

A   B

fig. 6.3. A. Erythrocytes in urine sediment. B. Leukocytes in urine sediment.

granules (see Figure 6.3). The granules will not be as apparent in the unstained urine as they would be if a supravital stain were used. Reduced lighting and fine focus adjustment while viewing will aid in identification of these cells. White blood cells are quantitated in the same manner as red blood cells.

Epithelial Cells. Epithelial cells line the urinary and genital tracts in multiple layers. The cells are constantly sloughed off or exfoliated and can be found in urine with regularity. Epithelial cells can be divided into three major types: **squamous, transitional,** and **renal** (see Figure 6.4). The type of cell found in the urine indicates the point of origin and determines the significance of the findings. Epithelial cells are summarized in Table 6.1.

Squamous epithelial cells are readily identified under low power and are the only epithelial cells which can be identified in this manner. They appear as large flat cells ranging in size from about 30 to 50 µm. The cells may be rectangular or round and sometimes appear irregular in shape due to folding or overlapping of multiple cells. The cells sometimes appear in "sheets." The nucleus is about the size of a red blood cell or small lymphocyte.

Transitional epithelial cells are round, oval, or variable in shape, depending on point of origin in the urinary tract. They are about 20 to 30 µm in diameter, with a distinctive nucleus. Renal epithelial cells are large, round cells and are not easily distinguished from transitional epithelial cells.

CASTS

Casts in the sediment result from protein being solidified in the kidney tubules. They are formed by either precipitation or conglutination (adherence) of materials in the tubule. Casts vary in structure. Additional material found in the tubule at the time of the protein solidification will be entrapped in the cast material. These materials include cells, bacteria, and fat.

The protein matrix that precipitates is a mucoprotein secreted only by the renal tubular cells. This matrix is known as the **Tamm-Horsfall protein.** The

Microscopic Examination of Urine

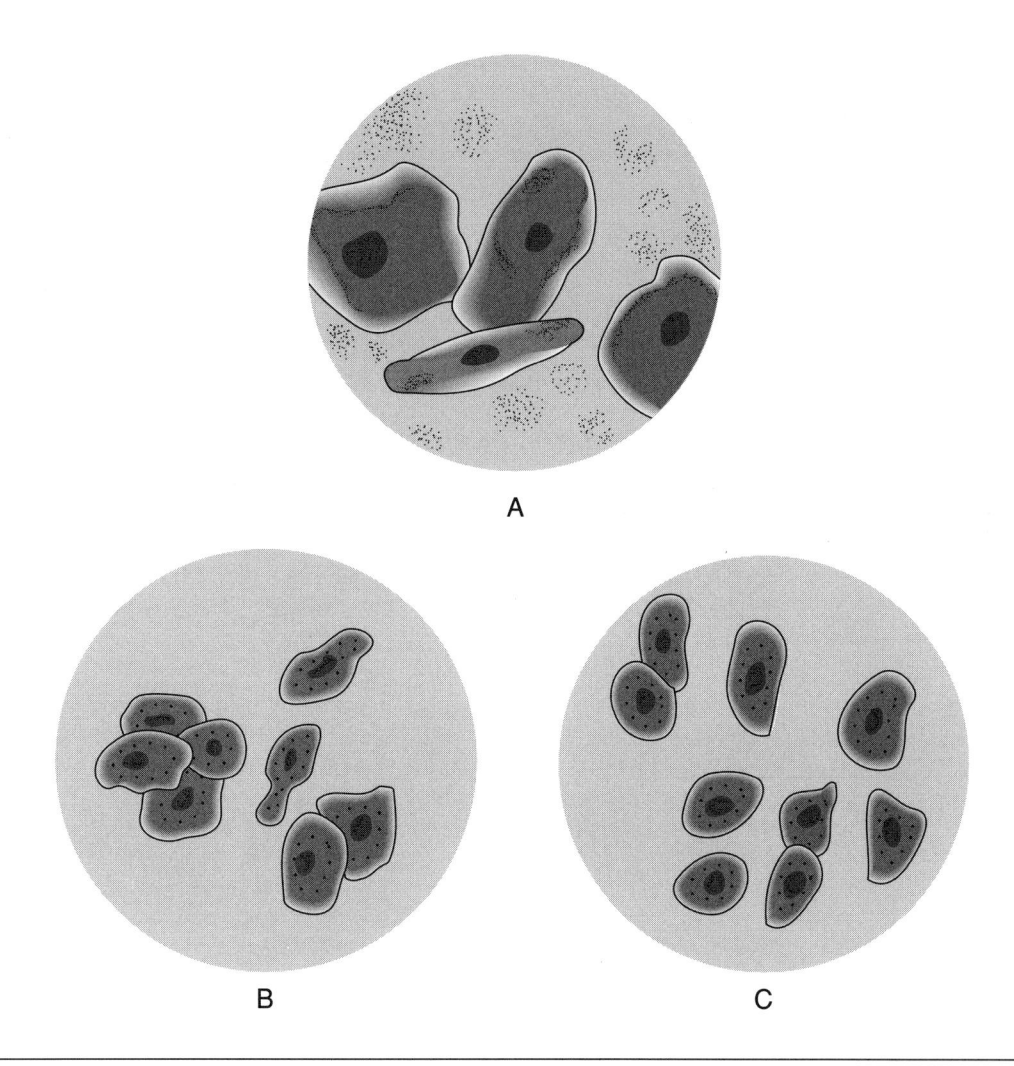

fig. 6.4. Epithelial cells in urine sediment. A. Squamous epithelial cells. B. Bladder epithelial cells. C. Renal epithelial cells.

Table 6.1. Epithelial Cells in Urine.

Squamous Epithelial Cells
Location: Lining of male and female urethra
Significance in Urine: Normal in small numbers
  Reflect an improperly collected or contaminated specimen in large numbers
Quantitation: Few, moderate, or many

Transitional Epithelial Cells
Location: Females—Lining of the urinary tract from the pelvis of the kidney to the base of the bladder
  Males—Lining of the urinary tract as in females but extending into the urethra
Significance in urine: Normal in small numbers
  Indicates urinary tract infection (UTI) or other clinical condition in large numbers
Quantitation: Few, moderate, or many

Renal Epithelial Cells
Location: Lining of the nephron tubules
Signification: Indicates renal disease
Quantitation: Few, moderate, or many

protein precipitates in the cylindrical shape of the tubules. The thickness and length will vary, as will the makeup of each individual cast.

Casts are quantitated by averaging the number per low power field. A numerical range is reported, *e.g.*, 0–2 or 2–4.

Hyaline Casts. Hyaline casts are the most commonly observed and insignificant of all the cast types. One or two may be found in the urine of normal, healthy individuals. Increased numbers of hyaline casts may be seen in the urine of individuals with physiological conditions such as dehydration, strenuous exercise, or fever. Hyaline casts are cylindrical in shape, with rounded ends (see Figure 6.5). They have a colorless, transparent appearance with a low refractive index that makes them difficult to visualize.

Granular Casts. Granular casts are composed of Tamm-Horsfall protein with degenerating cellular material in the matrix. The coarseness of the granularity of the casts is dependent on the stage of degeneration of the cellular material. These casts are classified as finely or coarsely granular (see Figure 6.5). As the degeneration is complete, these casts become a waxy cast.

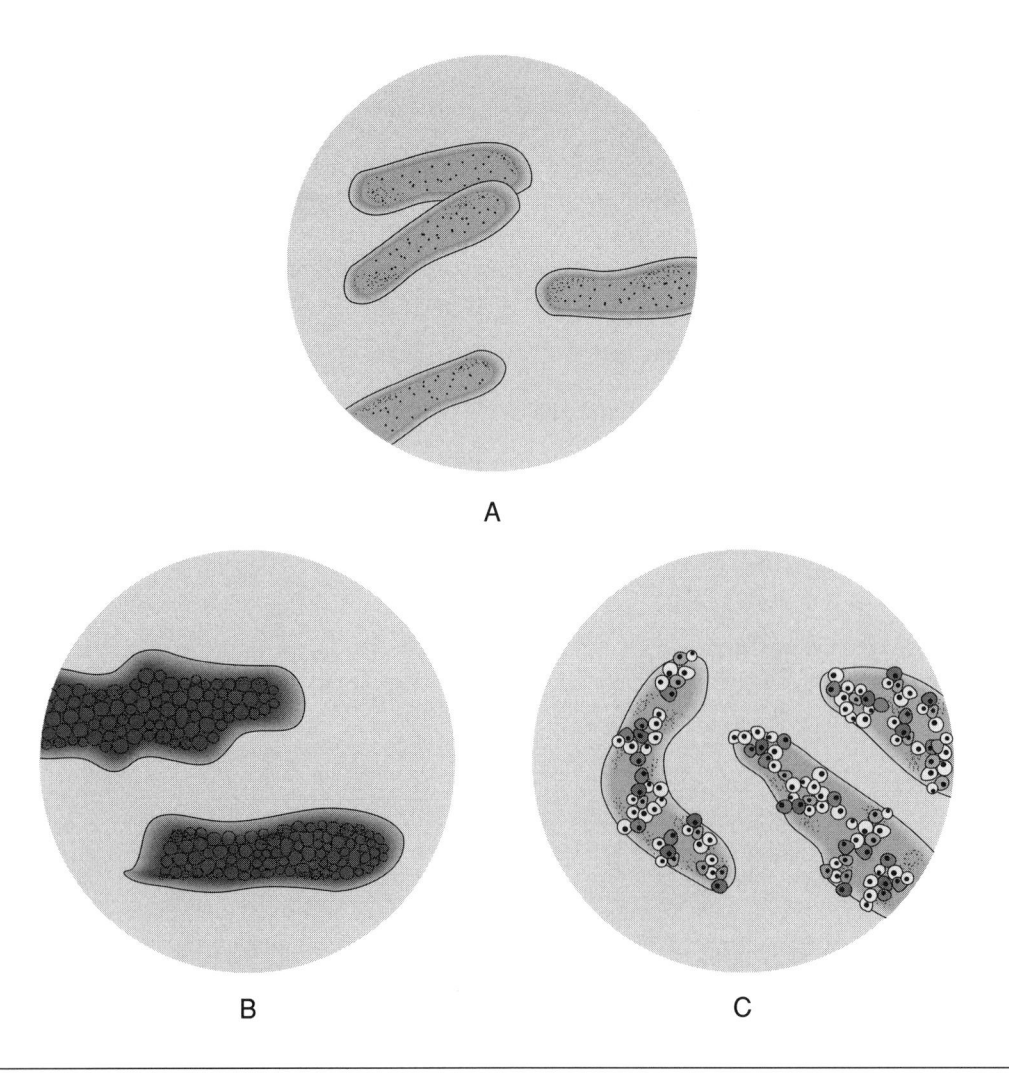

fig. 6.5. Casts in urine sediment. A. Hyaline casts. B. Granular casts. C. Cellular casts.

Granular casts are representative of glomerular injury and renal tubular damage. An occasional granular cast may be seen after strenuous exercise.

White Blood Cell Casts. White blood cell, or leukocyte, casts represent one form of cellular inclusion cast. As with the casts above, the cellular material is embedded in the Tamm-Horsfall protein. Presence of these casts in the urine represents an abnormal finding. It most often represents a sign of infection or inflammation. The leukocytes are usually phagocytic neutrophils. When examining the cast, it may appear as many cells tightly packed or a few cells scattered throughout the cast (see Figure 6.5). Compared to hyaline casts, white blood cell casts are relatively easy to visualize.

Red Blood Cell Casts. As with the white cell cast, the red cell cast is a hyaline cast with red cells embedded in the matrix (see Figure 6.5). These casts are fragile and disintegrate in old or stored urine. If the intact red cells are no longer present in the cast, it will appear as a brownish granular cast and should be called a hemoglobin or blood cast.

Red blood cell or blood casts are clinically significant and represent pathology in the nephron. These casts may be found in conditions such as glomerulonephritis, pyelonephritis, renal trauma, and others.

Epithelial Cell Casts. These are casts rarely seen in the urine. The presence of epithelial cell casts may imply renal disease or exposure to toxic substances or viruses. These casts vary in size, shape, and stage of degeneration (see Figure 6.5).

Waxy Casts. Waxy casts frequently appear with granular casts. They result from degeneration of granular casts. Waxy casts are homogenous in appearance with irregular and sometimes broken ends and edges. They are wider than hyaline casts and are easier to visualize and tend to have a high refractive index. Waxy casts appear yellow or grey in color. They are pathologically significant and often found in cases of severe renal failure.

Fatty Casts. Fatty casts contain fat droplets or **oval fat bodies.** Oval fat bodies consist of renal tubular epithelial cells or macrophages with ingested fat. These casts represent a clinically significant finding. They are found in cases of nephrotic syndrome, toxic nephrosis, and diabetes mellitus with renal degeneration. The fat appears to be light yellow or brown.

CRYSTALS

Crystals are not usually found in freshly voided urine. Rarely are crystals pathological. The formation of crystals is dependent on concentration of the solute, pH of the urine, and rate of urine flow through the tubules. Urinary crystals are summarized in Table 6.2.

Crystals are quantitated by specific type and counted as an average per low power field. The crystals are reported as a numerical range. Crystals will be categorized as appearing in acid or alkaline urines. It should be noted that some of these crystals may also be found in neutral urine (see Table 6.2).

▪ Unit 6

Crystals in Acid Urine. Crystals in acid urines are encountered at a pH of 6.5 or less. Many of the elements found in the acidic urines may be dissolved in alkaline conditions.

Amorphous urates appear as shapeless yellow-red or yellow-brown granules (see Figure 6.6). They impart an amber color and a fluffy precipitate appearance to the urine. They are composed of urate salts of sodium, potassium, magnesium, and calcium and have no clinical significance.

Uric acid crystals vary in shapes, with the most frequent shape being the diamond or rhombic prism (see Figure 6.7). They are seen commonly in urine and may be associated with gout when the serum uric acid level is also elevated.

Calcium oxalate is another frequently encountered crystal in the acid urine. They have a characteristic "envelope" appearance (see Figure 6.8). The crystals are actually an octahedral (eight-sided) shape and appear as small squares with an "X" or cross in the center. They are seen in the urine of normal individuals, and their appearance is frequently related to dietary constituents.

Cystine crystals are colorless hexagonal plates with either equal or unequal sides (see Figure 6.9). They are always significant and are associated with congenital disorders and the formation of calculi.

Table 6.2. Crystals Found in Urinary Sediment.

Crystals	pH	Microscopic appearance
Ammonium biurate	Alkaline or neutral	Yellow-brown striated spheres may have spicules
Amorphous phosphate	Alkaline or neutral	Colorless granules
Amorphous urates	Acid or neutral	Colorless or yellow-brown granules
Calcium carbonate	Alkaline or neutral	Colorless spheres or dumbbell shapes
Calcium oxalate	Acid or neutral	Colorless, octahedral or envelope shape
Calcium phosphate	Alkaline or neutral	Colorless granular plates or prism shapes
Cholesterol	Acid	Colorless, flat rectangle plates with notched corners
Cystine	Acid	Colorless, hexagonal plates sometimes layered
Leucine	Acid	Yellow-brown spheres, may have striations
Triple phosphates	Alkaline or neutral	Colorless, three- to six-sided prisms; "coffin lids"
Tyrosine	Acid	Colorless or yellow needles may be some clusters or sheaves
Uric acid		Colorless, yellow, or brown in many shapes may be layered

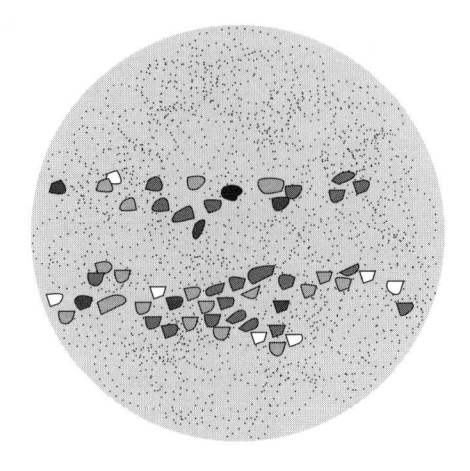

fig. 6.6. Amorphous urates/phosphates in urine sediment.

Microscopic Examination of Urine ▪

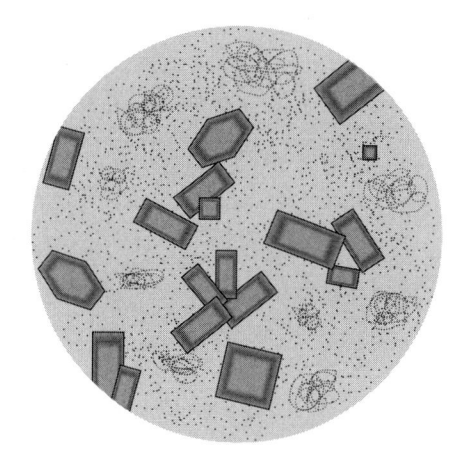

fig. 6.7. Uric acid crystals in urine sediment.

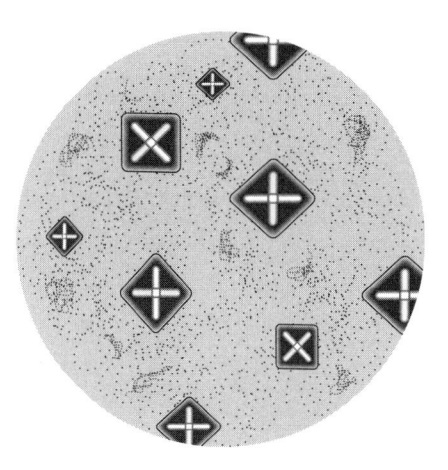

fig. 6.8. Calcium oxalate crystals in urine sediment.

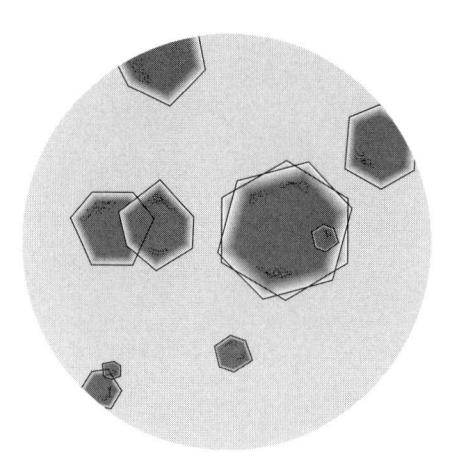

fig. 6.9. Cystine crystals in urine sediment.

Unit 6

Leucine crystals are highly refractile yellow or brown sphere-shaped crystals (see Figure 6.10). They may have visible radial striations. These crystals are very significant. They may be found in the urine of patients with maple syrup urine disease as well as in those with liver disease.

Tyrosine crystals appear needle-shaped in sheaves or clusters (see Figure 6.11). These needle shapes are highly refractile and readily seen with light microscopy. These crystals are found in rare metabolic disorders and liver disease.

Cholesterol crystals are large transparent plates with corners that appear notched (see Figure 6.12). They indicate an abundance of cholesterol in the urine and may appear with fat droplets, fatty casts, or oval fat bodies. These crystals may be seen in nephrotic syndrome as well as in conditions resulting in the rupture of lymphatic vessels into the renal tubules.

Medications and diagnostic substances of **iatrogenic** origin, such as ampicillin, sulfonamides, and radiographic contrast media, appear in the urine as crystalline substances. It is necessary to differentiate these substances from crystals with clinical significance.

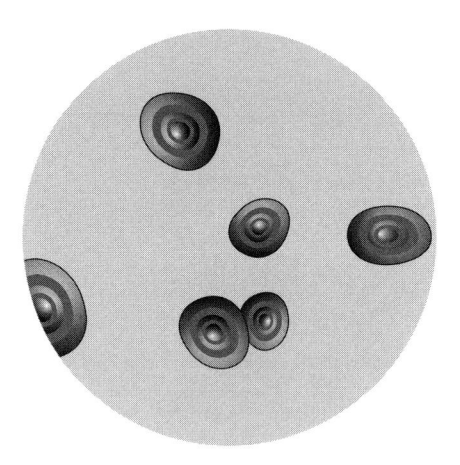

fig. 6.10. Leucine crystals in urine sediment.

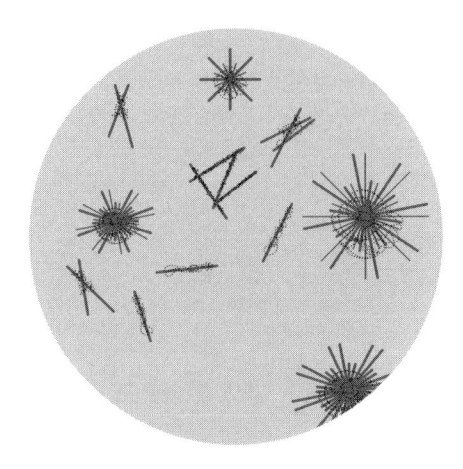

fig. 6.11. Tyrosine crystals in urine sediment.

Microscopic Examination of Urine

Crystals in Alkaline Urine. These crystals are found at a pH of 7.0 or higher and are frequently composed of phosphate or calcium. **Amorphous phosphates** are encountered in alkaline urine. They are indistinguishable from amorphous urates (see Figure 6.6) and have no clinical significance. Refrigeration of urines not examined within 2 hours will decrease the likelihood of deposition of these substances.

Triple phosphate crystals are encountered in alkaline urine. They are shaped as three- to six-sided prisms and may be described as coffin lids (see Figure 6.13). These crystals are found in the urine of normal individuals. They may contribute to the formation of calculi and be associated with some pathologic conditions such as pyelitis and chronic cystitis.

Calcium phosphate crystals are colorless and uncommon in normal urines. They may take many morphologic forms such as prisms with one pointed end. The prisms may be arranged as rosettes or stars, or they may appear as needles. These crystals may also form large, thin sheets or plates that may float on the top of the urine. They have little clinical significance.

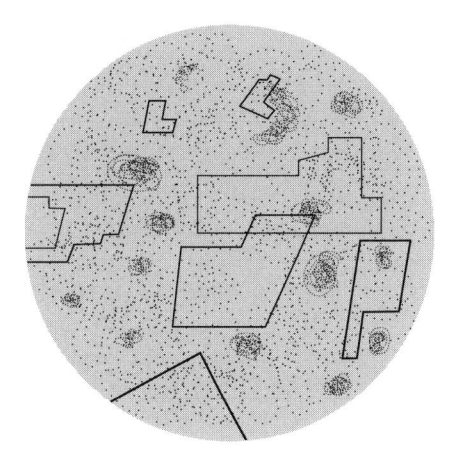

fig. 6.12. Cholesterol crystals in urine sediment.

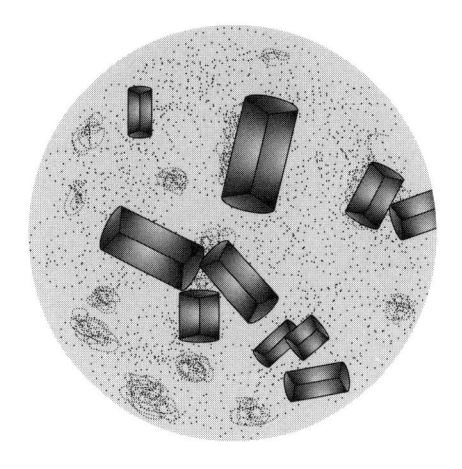

fig. 6.13. Triple phosphate crystals in urine sediment.

▪ Unit 6

Calcium carbonate crystals give the appearance of small, colorless granular crystals. They have a dumbbell appearance and may be in pairs. These crystals may be confused with amorphous material or bacteria. They have no clinical significance.

Ammonium biurate crystals are crystals with a spherical appearance. They appear yellow-brown in color and may have irregular projections that give them a "thorny-apple" appearance. These crystals frequently appear in urines that have been stored for a long period of time. When encountered in a urine, the collection and storage of that urine should be considered suspect and should be investigated. These crystals have no clinical significance.

Additional Morphological Structures

Additional structures that may be encountered in urine include bacteria, yeast, spermatozoa, mucus, and fat. These substances may be contaminants or may have a clinical significance, dependent upon the finding.

Bacteria. The observation of bacteria requires the use of the high-power objective. Bacteria may be rod shaped (bacilli) or round (coccoid). They are usually quantitated as few, moderate, or many. Their motility (movement) will distinguish them from amorphous substances.

When seen in significant numbers and in combination with white cells, bacteria indicate infection. Bacteria may be contaminants from vaginal or gastrointestinal areas or from the skin surrounding the urethral outlet. In these cases, the number present will be less than seen in infections. Keep in mind, however, that bacteria will multiply rapidly in urines that are improperly stored.

Yeast. Yeast in the urine may be contaminants from the vagina and the skin. Yeast has a characteristic oval, refractile, colorless appearance and may have buds (see Figure 6.14). Yeast may be confused with red cells but is smaller; the presence of buds will aid in this distinction.

Spermatozoa. Spermatozoa may be found in the urine of both sexes. They can be recognized by their oval bodies and long, thin, delicate tails. They are clinically insignificant.

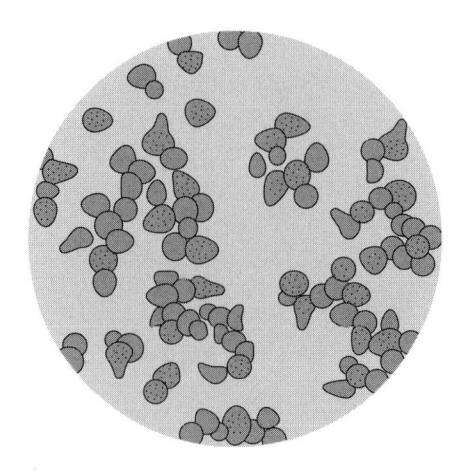

fig. 6.14. Yeast cells in urine sediment.

Microscopic Examination of Urine

Mucus. Mucus threads are very fine threads with a low refractive index. They are difficult to identify with brightfield microscopy. They are found in small numbers in normal urine and are more prevalent in women than in men. They tend to increase with inflammation or irritation of the urinary tract. In general, they have no clinical significance. They are composed of protein. The larger threads need to be differentiated from hyaline casts.

Fat. Fat in the urine presents as free droplets, globules, or oval fat bodies. Oval fat bodies are usually renal tubular cells with refractile fat droplets. They may also be white blood cells that have ingested lipids. The fat droplets appear refractile and are frequently yellow-brown in appearance. When present in high concentrations, these droplets may float on the surface of the urine.

Parasites. Occasionally parasites such as *Trichomonas vaginalis* and *Schistosoma* species may be seen in urine. If parasites are suspected, a current text on parasitology should be consulted.

Artifacts. Some items that are present in the microscopic urine did not originate in the urinary tract. These are contaminants and represent artifacts in the urinary sediment. Some examples of artifacts are fibers, hair, talc crystals, fat, oil, and pollen (see Figure 6.15).

PROCEDURE FOR MICROSCOPIC EXAMINATION OF URINE

Microscopic examination of urine requires the use of a fresh urine that is centrifuged and the sediment examined. The centrifugation concentrates the sediment in a range of 12:1 to 30:1. This concentration accounts for the ability to quantitate the formed elements seen. (See Table 6.3 for a system to quantitate formed elements in the concentrated urine.)

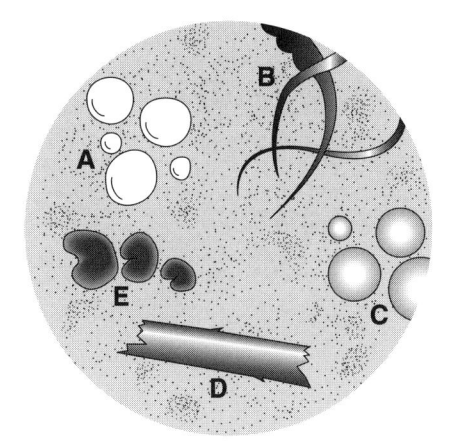

fig. 6.15. Common artifacts in urine sediment. A. Air bubbles. B. Fibers. C. Oil droplets. D. Hair. E. Starch granules.

• Unit 6

EXERCISE 36 REPORTING MICROSCOPIC URINALYSIS

Using sample urine report forms provided by the instructor, each student should:

1. Determine the ranges for reporting microscopic elements.
2. Compare the ranges used in different laboratories.
3. Discuss the findings in small groups.

Table 6.3. Quantitation of Urinary Sediment Elements.

Averge number per low power fields
System to Quantitate: Abnormal crystals
                     Casts
Scoring: Negative 0–2 2–5 5–10 10–25 25–50 >50
System to Quantitate: Squamous epithelial cells
Scoring: Few Moderate Many
System to Quantitate: Mucus
Scoring: Present

Average number per high power field
System to Quantitate: Red blood cells
                     White blood cells
Scoring: 0–2 2–5 5–10 10–25 25–50 50–100 >100
System to Quantitate: Normal crystals
                     Epithelial cells
                     Bacterial and yeast
Scoring: Few Moderate Many
System to Quantitate: Sperm (males only)
Scoring: Present

Most frequently, light microscopy is used and no stains are employed. Bearing this in mind, the following procedure should be used for each student to examine three urinary sediments:

EXERCISE 37 MICROSCOPIC EXAMINATION OF URINE

Equipment and supplies:

Microscope
Centrifuge
Conical tube

EXERCISE 37: MICROSCOPIC EXAMINATION OF URINE
continued

Test tube rack
Transfer pipettes
3- x 1-inch glass slides
Cover glass
Marking pen
Urine container and lid
Gloves
Goggles
Lab coat
Face shield
Puncture-proof biohazard container

NOTE: Gloves and other barrier protection should be worn throughout the urinalysis procedure.

Procedure:

1. Collect a midstream, clean catch urine sample.
2. Wearing gloves, goggles, lab coat, and face shield, perform all physical, chemical, and confirmatory tests. Record results.
3. Mix the urine specimen and decant approximately 12 ml into a conical centrifuge tube. Cap the specimen.
4. Centrifuge the capped specimen at 2000 rpm for 5 minutes.
5. Remove tubes from the centrifuge and decant most of the supernatant into a biohazardous waste receptacle or pour into the sink with copious amounts of water.
6. Mix the sediment to resuspend it in the remaining urine.
7. Transfer a drop to the slide using the transfer pipette.
8. Place the cover glass over the urinary sediment.
9. Allow to stand for 1 minute to permit settling of elements.
10. Place slide on microscope stage.
11. Using the 10x objective and reduced light, scan ten fields.
12. Look for crystals, casts, and cells and take a general overview of the contents.

NOTE: Be sure to examine near the edge of the cover glass, since casts tend to be pushed to the edges.

13. Enumerate casts and crystals and average per low-power field. Each type of cast and crystal should be reported as a range, e.g., 0–2, 2–4, etc.
14. Switch to the 40x objective.

• Unit 6

EXERCISE 37 MICROSCOPIC EXAMINATION OF URINE
continued

15. Enumerate formed elements as follows:
    WBC/high power field (hpf)
    RBC/hpf
    Epithelial cells/hpf
    WBCs, RBCs, and epithelial cells should be reported as numerical ranges.

    Note presence of mucus, bacteria, and yeast.
        Mucus, bacteria, and yeast should be reported as slight, few, moderate, many, and marked.
16. Record results on worksheet provided.
17. Repeat the above steps with additional specimens.
18. Discard all biohazardous waste into a puncture-proof biohazard container.

SUMMARY

Microscopic urinalysis is an important diagnostic tool in laboratory science. Significant morphological findings help to confirm and support diagnoses of clinical conditions. Microscopic urinalysis helps to establish the status of renal pathology and monitor treatment of some clinical conditions. It is important to distinguish microscopic elements that are clinically significant. Quantitation varies with each laboratory but is important when establishing significance of microscopic items.

Accompanying identification of the microscopic elements, proper collection, and storage are paramount to the accurate assessment of urinary sediment. Correct processing and identification will produce accurate and precise results of the urinary sediment examination.

REVIEW QUESTIONS

1. An objective has the marking "40x." This means that it
   a. contains 40 lenses
   b. magnifies 40 times
   c. views at a distance of 40 mm
   d. combines with ocular to magnify 40 times

Microscopic Examination of Urine

2. The coarse adjustment is used only when
   a. sharpening focus
   b. using oil immersion
   c. ocular is 10x
   d. using low power objective
3. When a technician switches from low to high power, the slide is no longer in focus. The microscope is not
   a. of binocular type
   b. illuminated properly
   c. parfocal for these objectives
   d. adjusted for interpupillary distance
4. A student is performing microscopic urinalysis. The part of the microscope that will *not* be required for adjusting the illumination is
   a. condenser
   b. iris diaphragm
   c. light source
   d. revolving nosepiece
5. In order to concentrate a urine for microscopic examination, the technician will treat the urine by
   a. centrifuging
   b. mixing
   c. shaking
6. The crystals found in acid urine are
   a. amorphous phosphates
   b. cholesterol
   c. calcium carbonate
   d. triple phosphate
7. The type of cast made entirely of Tamm-Horsfall protein is
   a. cellular
   b. granular
   c. hyaline
   d. waxy
8. Granular casts degenerate into
   a. cellular casts
   b. fatty casts
   c. hyaline casts
   d. waxy casts
9. Crystals which have a characteristic envelope appearance are
   a. ammonium biurate
   b. calcium carbonate
   c. calcium oxalate
   d. uric acid
10. When reporting casts they are reported as
    a. few, moderate, many, or marked per high power field
    b. few, moderate, many, or marked per low power field
    c. a numerical range per high power field
    d. a numerical range per low power field

UNIT 7

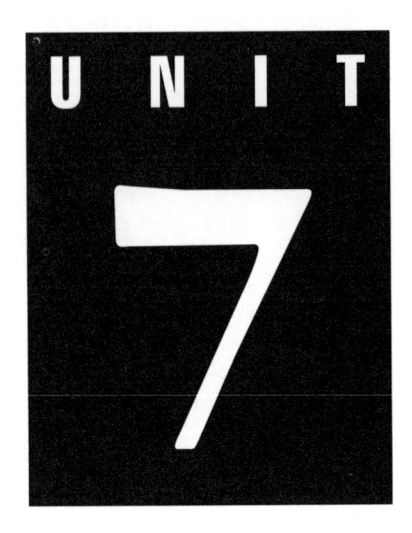

Case Studies in Urinalysis

LEARNING OBJECTIVES

After studying this unit, it is the responsibility of the student to know the following objectives:

- Analyze urinalysis data.
- Understand the interrelationship between the various tests.
- Be able to answer questions related to the data provided.

INTRODUCTION

The purpose of this unit is to give the student the chance to combine and synthesize material that was covered in the previous units. The case studies will require the student to review and analyze laboratory data obtained from a urinalysis. Questions for analysis that are related to the data will compel them to integrate previously learned material.

CASE STUDY NUMBER 1

BACKGROUND

A 12-year-old boy was examined in the emergency room. His mother said he was having frequent urination lasting several days. He was also complaining of feeling weak and tired.

PHYSICAL EXAMINATION

Color	Pale yellow
Clarity	Clear

CHEMICAL ANALYSIS

pH	6.0
Specific gravity	1.025
Protein	Trace
Glucose	1000 mg/dl
Ketone	5 mg/dl
Nitrite	Negative
Blood	Negative
Bilirubin	Negative
Urobilinogen	Negative
Leukocyte	Negative

MICROSCOPIC

RBC	0–2
WBC	0–2
Bacteria	Few
Epithelial cells	Few

OTHER TESTS

SSA	Trace

QUESTIONS

1. Which results are outside the normal range?
2. Based on these results, what might be the diagnosis?
3. What is the relationship between the appearance of ketones in urine and carbohydrate metabolism?

CASE STUDY NUMBER 2

BACKGROUND

A patient visits the doctor complaining of chronic pain near the bottom of his rib cage. The doctor collects a urine sample and asks the patient to submit a stool specimen as soon as possible. The patient returns the next day with a stool specimen that is very pale in color.

PHYSICAL EXAMINATION

Color	Amber
Clarity	Clear

CHEMICAL ANALYSIS

pH	6.0
Specific gravity	1.015
Protein	Trace
Glucose	Negative
Ketone	Negative
Nitrite	Negative
Blood	Negative
Bilirubin	Moderate
Urobilinogen	Normal
Leukocyte	Negative

MICROSCOPIC

RBC	0–2
WBC	0–2
Bacteria	Negative
Epithelial cells	None

OTHER TESTS

SSA	Trace

QUESTIONS

1. Which results are outside the normal range?
2. Is it likely that the urobilinogen is actually normal?
3. What is the significance, if any, of the stool specimen?

CASE STUDY NUMBER 3

BACKGROUND

A 23-year-old woman went to her doctor complaining of a burning sensation when urinating. She also commented that the urine was cloudy and had an unpleasant odor. The doctor ordered a urinalysis.

PHYSICAL EXAMINATION

Color	Yellow
Clarity	Cloudy

CHEMICAL ANALYSIS

pH	6.0
Specific gravity	1.018
Protein	30.0 mg/dl
Glucose	Negative
Ketone	Negative
Nitrite	Positive
Blood	Small
Bilirubin	Negative
Urobilinogen	Normal
Leukocyte	Positive

MICROSCOPIC

RBC	0–2
WBC	10–20
Bacteria	Many
Epithelial cells	Many

OTHER TESTS

SSA	30.0 mg/dl

QUESTIONS

1. What is the most probable diagnosis?
2. What follow-up tests may be ordered?
3. Are there any discrepancies between any of the test results?

• Unit 7

CASE STUDY NUMBER 4

BACKGROUND

A 2-week-old infant was brought to the emergency room. His mother said that he had had diarrhea and occasional vomiting since birth. In the last day he had developed jaundice. A urine specimen was collected.

PHYSICAL EXAMINATION

| Color | Yellow |
| Clarity | Clear |

CHEMICAL ANALYSIS

pH	6.5
Specific gravity	1.018
Protein	Negative
Glucose	Negative
Ketone	Negative
Nitrite	Negative
Blood	Negative
Bilirubin	Negative
Urobilinogen	Normal
Leukocyte	Negative

MICROSCOPIC

RBC	0–2
WBC	0–2
Bacteria	Few
Epithelial cells	Few

OTHER TESTS

| SSA | Not tested |
| Clinitest | 500 mg/dl |

QUESTIONS

1. Why is the reagent strip test for glucose negative and the Clinitest positive?
2. What condition is associated with these results?
3. If left untreated, what is the prognosis for the infant?

CASE STUDY NUMBER 5

BACKGROUND

A urine specimen was received in the laboratory as part of a transfusion reaction investigation. The following results were obtained.

PHYSICAL EXAMINATION

Color	Slightly pink
Clarity	Clear

CHEMICAL ANALYSIS

pH	5.0
Specific gravity	1.019
Protein	Trace
Glucose	Negative
Ketone	Negative
Nitrite	Negative
Blood	Small
Bilirubin	Moderate
Urobilinogen	2 mg/dl
Leukocyte	Negative

MICROSCOPIC

RBC	0
WBC	0–2
Bacteria	None
Epithelial cells	Few

OTHER TESTS

SSA	Trace

QUESTIONS

1. Why is the bilirubin negative while the urobilinogen is positive?
2. Why are no RBCs present in the microscopic examination while there was blood detected with the reagent strip?
3. Are there any clinical conditions that would give the same results? What are they?

CASE STUDY NUMBER 6

BACKGROUND

A 65-year-old man was admitted through the emergency room for treatment of a broken hip. Below are his urinalysis results.

PHYSICAL EXAMINATION

Color	Yellow
Clarity	Cloudy

CHEMICAL ANALYSIS

pH	5.0
Specific gravity	1.021
Protein	Negative
Glucose	Negative
Ketone	Negative
Nitrite	Negative
Blood	Negative
Bilirubin	Negative
Urobilinogen	Normal
Leukocyte	Negative

MICROSCOPIC

RBC	0–2
WBC	0–2
Bacteria	Few
Epithelial cells	Few

OTHER TESTS

SSA	3+

QUESTIONS

1. What condition is consistent with these results?
2. Why is there a discrepancy between the reagent strip test and the SSA?
3. What other testing would be done to confirm this condition?
4. What factors would cause false-positive results for the SSA test?

CASE STUDY NUMBER 7

BACKGROUND

A patient was admitted to the hospital complaining of severe lower back pain, especially when urinating. A urinalysis revealed the following results.

PHYSICAL EXAMINATION

Color	Red
Clarity	Cloudy

CHEMICAL ANALYSIS

pH	8.0
Specific gravity	1.025
Protein	Trace
Glucose	Negative
Ketone	Negative
Nitrite	Negative
Blood	Large
Bilirubin	Negative
Urobilinogen	Normal
Leukocyte	Negative

MICROSCOPIC

RBC	Too numerous to count
WBC	0
Bacteria	0
Epithelial cells	Few
Crystals	Calcium phosphate

OTHER TESTS

SSA	Trace

QUESTIONS

1. What condition is consistent with these results?
2. What is the significance of the pH?
3. Can diet modification help prevent a recurrence?

CASE STUDY NUMBER 8

BACKGROUND

A 15-year-old male was examined by his physician. He was complaining of frequent urination, constant thirst, and weakness. His urinalysis results were the following.

PHYSICAL EXAMINATION

Color	Colorless
Clarity	Clear

CHEMICAL ANALYSIS

pH	5.5
Specific gravity	1.003
Protein	Negative
Glucose	Negative
Ketone	Negative
Nitrite	Negative
Blood	Negative
Bilirubin	Negative
Urobilinogen	Normal
Leukocyte	Negative

MICROSCOPIC

RBC	0
WBC	0
Bacteria	0
Epithelial cells	Few

OTHER TESTS

SSA	Not done

QUESTIONS

1. What condition is consistent with constant urination?
2. Why is the specific gravity low?
3. Are there any discrepancies in the chemical tests?

CASE STUDY NUMBER 9

BACKGROUND

A 45-year-old woman was examined by her doctor as part of an annual physical. The doctor noted that she was very obese. A first morning urine specimen was submitted as part of the routine checkup. The following results were obtained.

PHYSICAL EXAMINATION

Color	Yellow
Clarity	Clear

CHEMICAL ANALYSIS

pH	5.0
Specific gravity	1.021
Protein	Negative
Glucose	Trace
Ketone	Negative
Nitrite	Negative
Blood	Negative
Bilirubin	Negative
Urobilinogen	Normal
Leukocyte	Negative

MICROSCOPIC

RBC	0–2
WBC	0–2
Bacteria	Few
Epithelial cells	Few

OTHER TESTS

SSA	Not done
Clinitest	Negative

QUESTIONS

1. Why is the reagent strip positive for glucose while the Clinitest is negative?
2. What condition may be developing in this patient?
3. How will test results change as time passes if this condition is left untreated?

- Unit 7

CASE STUDY NUMBER 10

BACKGROUND

A 29-year-old pregnant female of 32 weeks' gestation was admitted to the hospital. She complained of fever, nausea, lower back pain, and urgency and frequency of urination. She had noticed the inability to completely empty her bladder for about 2 weeks prior to this.

PHYSICAL EXAMINATION

Color	Yellow
Clarity	Cloudy

CHEMICAL ANALYSIS

pH	6.0
Specific gravity	1.006
Protein	1+
Glucose	Negative
Ketone	Negative
Nitrite	Positive
Blood	1+
Bilirubin	Negative
Urobilinogen	Normal
Leukocyte	Positive

MICROSCOPIC

RBC	Few
WBC	Many
Bacteria	Many
Epithelial cells	Few squamous; few renal tubular
Casts	Few: WBC, granular

OTHER TESTS

SSA	1+

QUESTIONS

1. What is the most likely diagnosis?
2. What is the significance of the microscopic elements in this patient?
3. How did pregnancy play a role in this condition?

SUMMARY

The purpose of this unit was to serve as a capstone for the manual. It enabled the student to correlate material from the preceding units. Prior to this, students concentrated on isolated subject matter without taking a broad view. However, case studies require the student to view the total informational picture and use judgment and reasoning to draw a conclusion.

The answers to these case studies can be found in Appendix B.

APPENDIX A • ANSWERS TO REVIEW QUESTIONS

UNIT 1 Formation of Urine

1. c
2. c
3. b
4. a
5. a
6. c
7. d
8. b
9. b
10. c

UNIT 2 Quality Control and Safety in the Urinalysis Laboratory

1. c
2. d
3. c
4. c
5. a
6. a
7. d
8. d
9. a
10. c

UNIT 3 Specimen Collection

1. b
2. d
3. d
4. a
5. b
6. c
7. b
8. a
9. c
10. a

UNIT 4 Physical Examination of Urine

1. a
2. d
3. c
4. a
5. c
6. d
7. b
8. b
9. b
10. b

UNIT 5 Chemical Examination of Urine

1. b
2. c
3. d
4. c
5. d
6. b
7. e
8. d
9. c
10. a
11. d
12. a
13. a
14. c
15. b

UNIT 6 Microscopic Examination of Urine

1. b
2. d
3. c
4. d
5. d
6. b
7. c
8. d
9. c
10. d

APPENDIX B • ANSWERS TO CASE STUDIES

CASE STUDY NUMBER 1

1. Protein, glucose, and ketone.
2. Diabetes mellitus.
3. Ketones appear in the urine when the body cannot effectively utilize carbohydrates. The body uses fat to maintain metabolism, and ketones are a breakdown product of fat metabolism.

CASE STUDY NUMBER 2

1. Bilirubin is the key irregular result as well as the pale stool specimen.
2. No, the urobilinogen is probably negative because of a biliary blockage (posthepatic obstruction) preventing bilirubin from entering the gastrointestinal tract. The dipstick, however, does not register negative for urobilinogen.
3. Urobilinogen is a compound that gives feces a dark color. Lack of urobilinogen will result in a pale stool specimen.

CASE STUDY NUMBER 3

1. Urinary tract/bladder infection.
2. A test to determine the type of bacteria and what antibiotics it is susceptible to. This test is called a culture and sensitivity.
3. Yes, the blood result on the dipstick and the microscopic blood. An explanation for not seeing more red blood cells while the dipstick is positive would be that the red blood cells are hemolyzed. Probably in this case a high bacterial presence will cause false-positive blood dipstick results.

CASE STUDY NUMBER 4

1. The dipstick will only detect glucose, whereas the Clinitest will detect any reducing substance.
2. Galactosemia, an inborn error of metabolism in which the patient cannot metabolize galactose.
3. Poor—mental retardation with early death.

CASE STUDY NUMBER 5

1. There is nothing wrong with the liver's ability to produce and excrete bilirubin. However, there is such a large amount of it being converted to urobilinogen because of the transfusion reaction that excess urobilinogen is appearing in the urine.
2. There are not intact red blood cells, only free hemoglobin.
3. Yes, see Table 5.5.

CASE STUDY NUMBER 6

1. Multiple myeloma.
2. The reagent strip test is sensitive primarily to albumin, whereas the SSA will detect all protein.
3. Protein electrophoresis.
4. High concentration of antibiotics, e.g., penicillin or radiographic dyes.

CASE STUDY NUMBER 7

1. Renal calculi.
2. Calculi form in alkaline pH.
3. Yes, a diet that will maintain an acidic urinary pH will help prevent a recurrence.

CASE STUDY NUMBER 8

1. Diabetes insipidus.
2. The urine is very dilute.
3. No, not for this condition.

CASE STUDY NUMBER 9

1. The reagent strip is more sensitive to glucose than the Clinitest.
2. Diabetes mellitus type II, usually noninsulin-dependent, generally can be controlled by diet.
3. Glucose would continue to rise.

CASE STUDY NUMBER 10

1. Acute pyelonephritis.
2. Bacteria indicates infection, whereas WBC casts indicate kidney involvement.
3. Pressure on the bladder that does not allow for complete emptying.

REFERENCES

Brunzel, N.A. *Fundamentals of Urine and Body Fluid Analysis*. Philadelphia: Saunders, 1994.

Graff, L. *A Handbook of Routine Urinalysis*. Philadelphia: Lippincott, 1983.

Hole, J.W., Jr. *Essentials of Anatomy and Physiology*. Dubuque, Iowa: William C. Brown, 1986.

Hundley, J.M. and Fleming, J.K. *Urine Analysis: Workshops in Medical Technology*. Chicago: ASCP, 1993.

Marshall, J. *Fundamental Skills for the Clinical Laboratory Professional*. Albany, N.Y.: Delmar, 1993.

Ringsrud, K.M. and Linne, J.J. *Urinalysis and Body Fluids: A Color Text and Atlas*. St. Louis: Mosby, 1995.

Strasinger, S.K. *Urinalysis and Body Fluids*, ed. 3, Philadelphia: F.A. Davis, 1994.

Walters, N.J., Estridge, B.H., and Reynolds, A.P. *Basic Medical Laboratory Techniques*. Albany, N.Y.: Delmar, 1990.

INDEX

Acetoacetic acid, 52
Acetone, 52
Acid urine, 48, 78-80, 81
Acid-base balance, formation of urine and, 8-9
Acidosis, metabolic, 52
Acquired immunodeficiency syndrome (AIDS), 18
Active transport, 7-8
ADH; see Antidiuretic hormone
Adherence, casts and, 74
AIDS; see Acquired immunodeficiency syndrome
Air bubbles in urine, 83
Albumin, 49
Aldosterone, ADH and, 10
Alkaline urine, 48, 81-82
Ames Multistix 10 reagent strip, 47, 55
Ames Multistix reagent strip, 47, 55
Ames N-Multistix reagent strip, 47, 55
Ammonium biurate crystals, 78, 82
Amorphous phosphates, 31, 38, 78, 81
   definition of, 36, 64
Amorphous urates, 31, 38, 78
   definition of, 36, 64
Antidiuretic hormone (ADH), 9-10
Appearance of urine, 38, 39
Artifacts in urine, 83
Ascorbic acid, false-negative reactions and, 51, 53, 54-55

Bacteria in urine, 82
Barrier protection, safety and, 19, 21
Bence-Jones protein, 56
Bicarbonate, acid-base balance and, 8
Bilirubin
   conjugated, 53
   definition of, 36
   in urine, 37, 53-56
Bilirubin confirmation test, 58
Binocular, definition of, 64
Binocular microscope, 65, 66
Biohazard label, 21

Biohazardous, definition of, 14
Biohazardous materials, 18-19, 20
Biological hazards, safety and, 18-19, 21
Bladder epithelial cells, 75
Bleach, biohazardous spills and, 19
Blood casts, 77
Blood in urine, 50-51
Boric acid as preservative, 31
Bowman's capsule, 4
   definition of, 2
Brightfield microscopy, 72
Bromthymol blue, 48

Calcium carbonate crystals, 78, 82
Calcium oxalate crystals, 78, 79
Calcium phosphate crystals, 78, 81
Calculi, 48
   definition of, 46
Calyx, 5
   definition of, 2
CAP; see College of American Pathologists
Capsule, Bowman's, 4
   definition of, 2
Carbohydrate, 52
   definition of, 46
Carbon dioxide, acid-base balance and, 8
Casts
   blood, 77
   cellular, 76
   epithelial cell, 77
   fatty, 77
   granular, 76-77
   hemoglobin, 77
   hyaline, 76
   leukocyte, 77
   red blood cell, 77
   in urine, 74-77
   waxy, 77
   white blood cell, 77
Cells in urine, 73-74
Cellular casts in urine, 76
Cellular components of urine, 3, 4
Centers for Disease Control, 18

Index

Chemical examination of urine, 45-62
Chemical hazards, safety and, 19-23
Chemical reagent strips; see Reagent strips
Chemical spill kit, 22-23
Chemical tests, 45-62
Chemstrip, 55
Chemstrip 7, 47
Chemstrip 8, 47
Chemstrip 9, 47
Chemstrip Automated Urine Analyzer, 59, 60
Chemstrip 10SG, 47
Cholesterol crystals, 78, 80, 81
Chromagen, 50
   definition of, 46
Clean catch midstream specimen, 29-30
   definition of, 27
Clinitest, 57
Coarse focus adjustments of microscope, 67
Collecting tubule, 5, 10
   definition of, 2
College of American Pathologists (CAP), 17
Color of urine, 37, 54
Concentration
   definition of, 2
   formation of urine and, 6, 9-10
Condenser, 68
   definition of, 64
Confirmatory tests of urine, 56-58, 59
Conglutination, casts and, 74
Conjugated bilirubin, 53
Containers
   specimen, 28, 29
   urine collection, 28, 29
Controls, lyophilized, 16
Convoluted tubule
   distal, 5
      definition of, 2
   proximal, 4
      definition of, 2
Copper reduction tests for sugar, 57-58
Cortex, 3, 4
   definition of, 2
Count 6 system, 72
Count 10 system, 72

Countercurrent, definition of, 2
Countercurrent mechanism, 9
Crenated cells, 73
Crystals, 77-83
   in acid urine, 78-80
   in alkaline urine, 81-82
Cystine crystals, 78, 79

Desiccant, 47
   definition of, 46
Diabetes insipidus, 39
   definition of, 36
Diabetes mellitus, 30, 53
   definition of, 27
Diaphragm, iris, 68
   definition of, 64
Diazonium salts, 54, 55
p-Dimethylaminobenzaldehyde, 55
Dipstick, 47
Distal convoluted tubule, 5
   definition of, 2
Diurnal, 29
   definition of, 27

Ehrlich's reagent, 55
Enzyme, 52
   definition of, 46
Epithelial cell casts, 77
Epithelial cells, 74, 75
   bladder, 75
   renal, 74, 75
      definition of, 64
   squamous, 72-73, 74, 75
      definition of, 64
   transitional, 74, 75
      definition of, 64
Erythrocytes, 74
Esterase, 52
External quality control, 18
   definition of, 14
Eyepiece of microscope, 65

False-negative reactions, 55
False-positive reactions, 55
Fasting, definition of, 27
Fasting specimen, 29
Fat bodies, oval, 77, 83
   definition of, 64
Fat droplets, 77, 83
Fat in urine, 83

Fatty casts in urine, 77
Fenestrated, definition of, 2
Fenestrated capillaries, 6
Fibers in urine, 83
Filtration
   definition of, 2
   formation of urine and, 6
Fine focus adjustments of microscope, 67
Fire drills, 23
Fire escape plans, 23
Fire extinguishers, 23
First morning specimen, 29, 32
   definition of, 27
Flammability, 21
   definition of, 14
Formaldehyde as preservative, 31
Formation of urine; see Urine, formation of
Formed elements in urinary sediment, 73-74

Galactosemia, 57
   definition of, 46
Galactosuria, 57
   definition of, 46
Glomerulonephritis, 39, 49
   definition of, 36, 46
Glomerulus, 4, 6
   definition of, 2
Gloves, soiled, removal of, 20
Glucose in urine, 53
Glucose oxidase, 53
Glucose tolerance test, 30, 32
   definition of, 27
Glucosuria, 53
   definition of, 46
Glycosuria, 53
   definition of, 46
Granular casts in urine, 76-77
Granulated leukocytes, 52
   definition of, 46
Granulocytes, 52

Hair in urine, 83
Handwashing techniques, 19
HBV; see Hepatitis B virus
Hematuria, 50, 73
   definition of, 46, 64

Hemoglobin, 37, 50
   definition of, 36, 46
   normal metabolism of, 54
Hemoglobin casts, 77
Hemoglobinuria, 50
   definition of, 46
Henle, loop of, 4-5
   definition of, 2
Hepatitis B virus (HBV), 18, 37
HIV; see Human immunodeficiency virus
Human immunodeficiency virus (HIV), 18
Hyaline casts in urine, 76
[beta]-Hydroxybutyric acid, 52
Hypersthenuria, 39
   definition of, 36
Hypertonic, 9
   definition of, 2
Hyposthenuria, 39
   definition of, 36

Iatrogenic, 80
   definition of, 64
Ictotest, 58
Illumination of microscope, 67-68
Instrument maintenance, quality control and, 17
Instrumentation, urinalysis, 58-60
Insulin, 52
Internal quality control, 18
   definition of, 14
Interpupillary distance, 65
   definition of, 64
Intravenous pyelogram, 39
Iris diaphragm, 68
   definition of, 64
Isotonic urine, 73

Jaundice, 53
   definition of, 46
JCAHO; see Joint Commission on Accreditation of Healthcare Organizations
Joint Commission on Accreditation of Healthcare Organizations (JCAHO), 17

Ketones in urine, 52-53
Ketosis, 52

Index

Kidney, 3-5
  cross section of, 4
  functions of, 6
Kidney stones, 48
Kova system, 72

Labeling, specimen, 28, 29
Legal's test, 52
Leucine crystals, 78, 80
Leukocyte casts, 77
Leukocytes, 52, 74
  granulated, 52
    definition of, 46
Light microscopy, 72
Light reflection, principle of, 60
Light source of microscope, 67-68
Loop of Henle, 4-5
  definition of, 2
Lymphocytes, 52
Lyophilized, definition of, 14
Lyophilized controls, 16

Magnification
  of microscope, 65-67
  total, 65-67
    definition of, 64
Malabsorption, ketones and, 52
Maple syrup urine disease, 42, 80
  definition of, 36
Material safety data sheet (MSDS), 21, 22
Medulla, 3
  definition of, 2
Metabolic acidosis, 52
Methyl red, 48
Microscope, 65-71
  binocular, 65, 66
  care of, 69, 70-71
  coarse and fine focus adjustments of, 67
  illumination of, 67-68
  magnification and, 65-67
  parts of, 65-68
  storage of, 70-71
  transporting of, 69
  use of, 65-71
Microscopic examination of urine, 63-87
  constituents of normal urine sediment in, 72-73
  formed elements in urinary sediment in, 73-74
  procedure for, 83-86
  specimen collection and handling in, 71-72
  standardization of, 72
  techniques of, 72
Microscopy
  brightfield, 72
  light, 72
  phase contrast, 72, 73
  polarizing, 72, 73
Midstream urine collection, 29, 32
  definition of, 27
Monocular, definition of, 64
Monocular microscope, 65
MSDS; see Material safety data sheet
Mucus threads in urine, 83
Multiple myeloma, 49
  definition of, 46
Myoglobin, 50
  definition of, 46

National Committee for Clinical Laboratory Standards, 17
National Fire Protection Association (NFPA), 19-21, 22, 23
Nephron, 4, 5
  absorption and secretion within, 7
  definition of, 2
  diagramming, 6
  physiologic functions of, 10
Neutrophils, phagocytic, 77
NFPA; see National Fire Protection Association
Nitrate, 51
Nitrite, 51
Nosepiece, revolving, 65
  definition of, 64

Objectives, 65
  definition of, 64
Occupational Safety and Health Administration (OSHA), 18
Ocular, 65
  definition of, 64
Odor of urine, 41-42
Oil droplets in urine, 83
Oil-immersion objective, 65, 67

Index

Opaque, 28
   definition of, 27
Orthostatic proteinuria, 49
   definition of, 46
   screening procedures for, 49
OSHA; *see* Occupational Safety and Health Administration
Osmotic gradient, 9
Oval fat bodies, 77, 83
   definition of, 64

Parasites in urine, 83
Parfocal, 67
   definition of, 64
Pass through reactions, 57
Passive transport, 7-8
Pelvis, renal, 5
   definition of, 2
Peritoneum, 3
   definition of, 2
pH of urine, 8, 48
Phagocytic neutrophils, 77
Phase contrast microscopy, 72, 73
Physical examination of urine, 35-44
Polarizing microscopy, 72, 73
Pooled urine specimen, 30
Postural proteinuria, 49
Precipitation, casts and, 74
Preservatives
   effect of, on urine, 31
   specimen collection and, 31-32
Procedure manuals, quality control and, 17
Protein, 49, 50
   Bence-Jones, 56
   Tamm-Horsfall, 49, 74-76
     definition of, 64
Protein Error of Indicators, 49
Protein precipitation test, 56-57
Protein reagent strip test results, 50
Protein sulfosalicylic acid precipitation test, 56, 57
Proteinuria, 49
   definition of, 46
   orthostatic; *see* Orthostatic proteinuria
   postural, 49
Proximal convoluted tubule, 4
   definition of, 2

Pyelogram
   definition of, 36
   intravenous, 39
Pyelonephritis, 39
   definition of, 36
Pyuria, 73
   definition of, 64

Quality assurance
   definition of, 14
   quality control and, 15
Quality control, 13-25
   definition of, 14
   external, 18
     definition of, 14
   instrument maintenance and, 17
   internal, 18
     definition of, 14
   procedure manuals and, 17
   quality assurance and, 15
   specimen collection and handling and, 15
   test performance and, 15-17

Random sample, 28-29
Random specimen, 32
   definition of, 27
Rapimat II, 60
Reabsorption
   definition of, 2
   formation of urine and, 6, 7-8
Reagent strips, 39, 41, 47-56, 54
   protein, results of, 50
Red blood cell casts in urine, 77
Red blood cells in urine, 50, 73, 74
Refractive index, 39
Refractometer, 39-41, 42
Refrigeration as preservative, 31
Removal of soiled gloves, 20
Renal epithelial cells, 74, 75
   definition of, 64
Renal pelvis, 5
   definition of, 2
Renal physiology, formation of urine and, 6-10
Renal structure, formation of urine and, 3-5
Renal threshold, 8
   definition of, 2

Index

Revolving nosepiece, 65
   definition of, 64

Safety equipment, location of, 23
Safety in urinalysis laboratory, 18-23
   barrier protection and, 19, 21
   biological hazards and, 18-19, 21
   chemical hazards and, 19-23
Safety procedure, 21
Schistosoma species in urine, 83
Secretion
   definition of, 2
   formation of urine and, 6, 8-9
Sediment, urinary; *see* Urinary sediment
Self-adhering labels, 28
Sodium fluoride as preservative, 31
Sodium hypochlorite solution, biohazardous spills and, 19
Soiled gloves, removal of, 20
Solutes in urine, 3
Specific gravity of urine, 38-41, 42, 56
   high, 39
   low, 38-39
Specimen collection, 26-34, 38
   containers and labeling and, 28, 29
   in microscopic examination of urine, 71-72
   preservatives and, 31-32
   quality control and, 15
   types of specimens and, 28-30
Spermatozoa in urine, 82
Squamous epithelial cells, 72-73, 74, 75
   definition of, 64
SSA precipitation test; *see* Sulfosalicylic acid precipitation test
Stain, supravital, 72
   definition of, 64
Standardization in microscopic examination of urine, 72
Starch granules in urine, 83
Starvation, ketones and, 52
Sulfosalicylic acid, 57
Sulfosalicylic acid (SSA) precipitation test, 56, 57
Supernatant, 71-72
Supplementary tests of urine, 56-58
Supravital stain, 72
   definition of, 64

Tamm-Horsfall protein, 49, 74-76
   definition of, 64
Test performance, quality control and, 15-17
Timed specimen, 30
   definition of, 27
Total magnification, 65-67
   definition of, 64
Transitional epithelial cells, 74, 75
   definition of, 64
Translucent, 28
   definition of, 27
Trichomonas vaginalis in urine, 83
Triple phosphate crystals, 78, 81
Turbid, 38
   definition of, 36
Twelve-hour urine collection, 32
Twenty-four-hour urine collection, 32
Two-hour postprandial specimen, 30, 32
   definition of, 27
Tyrosine crystals, 78, 80

Ultrafiltrate, 3, 6
   definition of, 2
Universal Precautions, 18, 37
   definition of, 14
Uric acid crystals, 48, 78, 79
Urinalysis instrumentation, 58-60
Urinalysis laboratory, quality control and safety in, 13-25
Urinary constituents, 3
Urinary sediment, 71-72
   definition of, 64
   formed elements in, 73-74
   normal, constituents of, 72-73
   quantitation of elements of, 84
Urinary tract infection (UTI), 51, 52
Urine
   acid, 48, 78-80, 81
   alkaline, 48, 81-82
   appearance of, 38, 39
   artifacts in, 83
   bacteria in, 82
   bilirubin confirmation test of, 58
   bilirubin in, 53-56
   blood in, 50-51

Index

casts in, 74-77
cells in, 73-74
cellular components of, 4
chemical examination of, 45-62
color of, 37, 54
composition of, 3
confirmatory tests of, 56-58, 59
copper reduction tests for sugar in, 57-58
crystals in, 77-83
epithelial cell casts in, 77
epithelial cells in, 74, 75
fat in, 83
fatty casts in, 77
formation of, 1-12
  acid-base balance and, 8-9
  concentration and, 6, 9-10
  filtration and, 6
  reabsorption and, 6, 7-8
  renal physiology and, 6-10
  renal structure and, 3-5
  secretion and, 6, 8-9
glucose in, 53
granular casts in, 76-77
hyaline casts in, 76
instrumentation in examination of, 58-60
ketones in, 52-53
leukocytes in, 52
microscopic examination of; *see* Microscopic examination of urine
mucus in, 83
nitrite in, 51
odor of, 41-42
parasites in, 83
pH of, 48
physical examination of, 35-44
protein in, 49, 50
protein precipitation test of, 56-57
reagent strips in examination of, 47-56
red blood cell casts in, 77
red blood cells in, 73, 74
sediment of; *see* Urinary sediment
specific gravity of, 38-41, 42, 56
spermatozoa in, 82
substances eliminated through, 8
supplementary tests of, 56-58
urobilinogen in, 53-56
waxy casts in, 77
white blood cells casts in, 77
white blood cells in, 73-74
yeast in, 82
Urine collection containers, 28, 29
Urine control values, 17
Urinometer, 39, 40, 42
UriSystem, 72
Urobilinogen in urine, 53-56
Urochrome, 37
  definition of, 36
UTI; *see* Urinary tract infection

Vitamin C, false-negative reactions and, 51

Waxy casts in urine, 77
White blood cells casts in urine, 77
White blood cells in urine, 73-74
Working distance, 67
  definition of, 64

Yeast in urine, 82